# THE *Skinny*
# ONE POT
## CASSEROLES & STEWS
### RECIPE BOOK

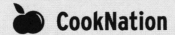

CookNation

# THE SKINNY ONE POT, CASSEROLES & STEWS RECIPE BOOK

Simple & Delicious, One-Pot Meals. All Under 300, 400 & 500 Calories.

**Copyright © Bell & Mackenzie Publishing Limited 2014**

**ISBN 978-1-909855-63-2**

A CIP catalogue record of this book is available from the British Library

## DISCLAIMER

Some recipes may contain nuts or traces of nuts. Those suffering from any allergies associated with nuts should avoid any recipes containing nuts or nut based oils.

This information is provided and sold with the knowledge that the publisher and author do not offer any legal or other professional advice.

In the case of a need for any such expertise consult with the appropriate professional.

This book does not contain all information available on the subject, and other sources of recipes are available.

This book has not been created to be specific to any individual's requirements.

Every effort has been made to make this book as accurate as possible. However, there may be typographical and or content errors. Therefore, this book should serve only as a general guide and not as the ultimate source of subject information.

This book contains information that might be dated and is intended only to educate and entertain.

The author and publisher shall have no liability or responsibility to any person or entity regarding any loss or damage incurred, or alleged to have incurred, directly or indirectly, by the information contained in this book.

# CONTENTS

# SKINNY ONE-POT VEGETABLE DISHES 47

# SKINNY ONE-POT SEAFOOD DISHES 65

# SKINNY HOMEMADE STOCK                                     **83**

# OTHER COOKNATION TITLES                                   **89**

# INTRODUCTION

*In every country and culture around the world there is a variation of the one-pot meal.*

In Spain a paella, France a boeuf bourguignon, a Moroccan tagine, Italian risotto or a classic Irish stew. Whatever the geography, the concept of cooking delicious meals with minimal preparation, maximum flavour and less cleaning up is a winning combination. Add to this mix carefully selected low calorie ingredients, which ensure each recipe falls below 300, 400 or 500 calories, and you have the perfect calorie controlled meal to help you manage your weight.

Whatever the dish used to prepare the meal - be it a casserole, tagine, wok or saucepan – all require just one-pot to blend flavours together, tenderising ingredients making a flavour packed, wholesome, nutritious and delicious meal that all the family can enjoy. One-pot dinners are much more than just meat and potatoes; our recipes include a wide selection of tasty choices including Sweet Pork & Beans and Creamy Butternut Squash Stew as well as some of the more classic dishes such as Northern Hot Pot and Beef & Guinness Stew.

One-pot meals are particularly good for week-night suppers. Quick to prepare, with no fuss they can be cooked and stored ahead of time ready to warm through for a hearty, perfectly balanced family meal. The combination of ingredients in many recipes makes it easy to include a selection of nutritious vegetables ensuring everyone gets part of their daily quota. Meal times don't get much heartier and simpler than one-pot meals.

When cooking our skinny one-pot meals you should follow these basic principles to achieve the best results:

## SAUCEPANS & CASSEROLES
Good quality dishes do achieve better results which can prevent your dishes from burning and sticking. Use heavy based saucepans and flameproof casserole dishes. Lids are often required for recipes so check before you start.

## MEAT
Browning meat is very important. You may be tempted to skip this part but the end results will be inferior if you do. Browning meat gives your dish both flavour and colour and by sealing in hot oil it retains its juices. Don't add too much meat to a saucepan when browning – it's better to brown in batches as a build up of steam in a crowded pan will inhibit the browning process.

Part of the joy of one-pot meals that require slower cooking is that tougher cuts of meat can be transformed into delicious and tender bites. The good news for the cook is that cheaper cuts of meat can therefore be used in many recipes.

Trim all meats of any excess fats. While certain cuts of meat such as chicken thighs may be suited to a one-pot recipe, these tend to be much higher in fat and calories so our skinny recipes opt for the leaner cuts of meat wherever possible.

## STOCK

Many of our skinny one-pot meals require a good stock as a base. There are many good quality stocks available in supermarkets so feel free to use these however be careful of the salt content. Not only is excessive salt not good for your health it can also ruin a dish. Alternatively you can use one of our homemade skinny stocks – see page 83 for the recipes.

## ABOUT COOKNATION

CookNation is the leading publisher of innovative and practical recipe books for the modern, health conscious cook.

CookNation titles bring together delicious, easy and practical recipes with their unique approach - making cooking for diets and healthy eating fast, simple and fun.

With a range of #1 best-selling titles - from the innovative 'Skinny' calorie-counted series, to the 5:2 Diet Recipes collection - CookNation recipe books prove that 'Diet' can still mean 'Delicious'!

Turn to the end of this book to browse all CookNation's recipe books

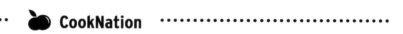 CookNation

# Skinny
# ONE POT
# MEAT
## DISHES

# SWEET PORK & BEANS

**375**
calories per serving

## Ingredients

- 2 onions, chopped
- 8 slices lean, back bacon, chopped
- 800g/1¾lb tinned cannellini beans, drained
- 1 tbsp brown sugar
- 2 tbsp tomato puree/paste
- 1 tbsp Dijon mustard
- 1 tbsp red wine vinegar
- 250ml/1 cup chicken stock
- Low cal cooking oil spray
- Salt & pepper to taste

## Method

**1** Preheat the oven to 180c/350f/Gas4

**2** Using a flameproof casserole dish gently sauté the onions and chopped bacon in a little low cal spray for a few minutes until softened (add a splash of water if it's a little dry).

**3** Add all the ingredients to the casserole dish, combine well and bring to a simmer. Cover, transfer to the preheated oven and cook for 1-1 ½ hours or until the stew is bubbling hot and cooked through.

**4** Check the stew during cooking. If it needs more liquid add a little stock. If you find there is too much, remove the lid and cook for a little longer to reduce the liquid.

**5** Check the seasoning and serve.

### CHEFS NOTE
You can use pre-soaked dried beans if you prefer but they'll need a little longer in the oven.

# SMOKED BLACK EYE BEAN & SAUSAGE STEW

495
calories per serving

## Ingredients

- 1 onion, chopped
- 2 garlic cloves, crushed
- 4 lean pork sausages
- 125g/4oz smoked gammon, finely chopped
- 1 tsp smoked paprika
- 2 tbsp tomato puree/paste
- 700g/1lb 9oz tinned black eye beans, drained
- 120ml/½ cup chicken stock
- Low cal cooking oil spray
- Salt & pepper to taste

## Method

**1** Using a flameproof casserole dish gently sauté the onions, garlic & pork sausages in a little low cal spray for a few minutes until the onions are softened and the sausages begin to brown (add a splash of water if it's a little dry).

**2** Remove the sausages and cut into 1cm/½ inch slices. Put all the ingredients back into the casserole dish and combine well. Bring to a hard simmer, cover, reduce the heat and leave to gently cook for 20-25 minutes or until the stew is piping hot and everything is cooked though.

**3** Check the stew during cooking. If it needs more liquid add a little stock. If you find there is too much, remove the lid and cook for a little longer to reduce the liquid.

**4** Use the back of a fork to gently mash some of the beans to give the stew a thicker consistency. Check the seasoning and serve.

## CHEFS NOTE

Chopped coriander makes a good garnish for this dish.

# SPICED LAMB & ALE STEW

**410** calories per serving

## Ingredients

- 1 red onion, chopped
- 1 white onion, chopped
- 4 garlic cloves, crushed
- 1 red chilli, deseeded & finely chopped
- 500g/1lb 2oz lean lamb fillet, cubed
- 1 tsp each ground cumin & coriander/cilantro

- 250ml/1 cup ale
- 1 tbsp balsamic vinegar
- 200g/7oz tinned chopped tomatoes
- 350g/12oz small new potatoes, halved
- Low cal cooking oil spray
- Salt & pepper to taste

## Method

**1** Using a flameproof casserole dish gently sauté the onions, garlic & chilli in little low cal spray for a few minutes until softened (add a splash of water if it's a little dry). Remove to a plate, add a little more oil to the casserole dish, increase the heat and quickly brown the lamb for a few minutes.

**2** Add all the ingredients, except the potatoes, back into the casserole dish and combine well. Bring to a hard simmer, cover, reduce the heat and leave to gently cook for 1 hour. Add the potatoes and continue to cook for 20-30 minutes or until the stew is piping hot, the potatoes are tender and the lamb is cooked though.

**3** Check the stew during cooking. If it needs more liquid add a little stock. If you find there is too much, remove the lid and cook for a little longer to reduce the liquid. Season and serve.

## CHEFS NOTE

You could replace the lamb with pork tenderloin if you like.

# FAMILY CHILLI

**480** calories per serving

## Ingredients

- 1 red onion, chopped
- 1 white onion, chopped
- 2 garlic cloves, crushed
- 1 red pepper, deseeded & sliced
- 1 tsp ground cumin
- 2 tbsp tomato puree/paste
- 400g/14oz tinned chopped tomatoes
- 2 tsp clear honey

- 400g/14oz tinned mixed beans, drained
- 600g/1lb 5oz lean beef mince/ground beef
- 2 sun dried tomatoes, finely chopped
- 120ml/½ cup beef stock
- Low cal cooking oil spray
- Salt & pepper to taste

## Method

**1** Preheat the oven to 180c/350f/Gas4

**2** Using a flameproof casserole dish gently sauté the onions, garlic & peppers in little low cal spray for a few minutes until softened (add a splash of water if it's a little dry). Remove to a plate, add a little more oil to the casserole dish, increase the heat and quickly brown the mince for a few minutes.

**3** Add all the ingredients back into the casserole dish and combine well. Bring to a hard simmer, cover and place in the preheated oven for 1–1½ hours or until the chilli is piping hot and the mince is cooked though.

**4** Check the chilli during cooking. If it needs more liquid add a little stock. If you find there is too much, remove the lid and cook for a little longer to reduce the liquid. Season and serve.

## CHEFS NOTE

This family friendly chilli doesn't contain any hot spice so you could add a little chilli powder if you like.

# BEEF & GUINNESS STEW

**470** calories per serving

## Ingredients

- 500g/1lb 2oz lean chuck steak, cubed
- 1 onion, chopped
- 1 leek, chopped
- 1 celery stalk, chopped
- 2 garlic cloves, crushed
- 2 large carrots, chopped
- 125g/4oz mushrooms, sliced

- 1 tbsp plain/all purpose flour
- 400g/14oz tinned chopped tomatoes
- 2 tbsp Worcestershire sauce
- 500ml/2 cups Guinness
- 1 tbsp Dijon mustard
- Low cal cooking oil spray
- Salt & pepper to taste

## Method

**1** Preheat the oven to 160c/325f/Gas3

**2** Using a flameproof casserole dish quickly brown the beef in a little low cal oil for a few minutes. Remove the beef, add a little more oil and gently sauté the onions, leek, celery, carrots, mushrooms & garlic for a few minutes until softened (add a splash of water if it's a little dry). Stir through the flour until well combined. Add the Worcestershire sauce, Guinness & mustard and cook for two minutes stirring throughout.

**3** Bring to the boil, cover and place in the preheated oven to cook for approximately 2 hours or until the beef is lovely and tender.

**4** Check the stew during cooking. If it needs more liquid add a little stock. If you find there is too much, remove the lid and cook for a little longer to reduce the liquid. Season and serve.

## CHEFS NOTE

This stew is lovely served with simple braised cabbage.

# NORTHERN STEW

**SERVES 4**

**460** calories per serving

## Ingredients

- 500g/1lb 2oz lean lamb fillet, cubed
- 2 onions, chopped
- 1 parsnip, chopped
- 2 large carrots, chopped
- 1 tbsp plain/all purpose flour
- 500ml/2 cups beef stock
- 150g/5oz peas
- 2 tsp marmite
- 2 tsp mixed dried herbs
- 500g/1lb 2oz potatoes, peeled & thinly sliced
- Low cal cooking oil spray
- Salt & pepper to taste

## Method

1 Preheat the oven to 160c/325f/Gas3

2 Using a flameproof casserole dish quickly brown the lamb in a little low cal oil for a few minutes. Remove the lamb, add a little more oil and gently sauté the onions, parsnips & carrots for a few minutes until softened (add a splash of water if it's a little dry). Stir through the flour until well combined. Add the stock and cook for two minutes stirring throughout.

3 Bring to the boil and remove from the heat. Place the sliced potatoes on top of the stew to create a potato topping. Spray with a little low cal oil, cover and place in the preheated oven to cook for approximately 2 hours or until the lamb & potatoes are cooked through and tender.

4 Remove the lid for the last half hour of cooking, season and serve.

### CHEFS NOTE
You may like to brown the potato topping under a hot grill for a few minutes just before serving..

# BARLEY & BEEF ONE-POT

**495**
calories per serving

## Ingredients

- 500g/1lb 2oz lean chuck steak, cubed
- 2 onions, chopped
- 1 celery stalk, chopped
- 1 garlic clove, crushed
- 2 large carrots, chopped
- 125g/4oz mushrooms, sliced
- 75g/3oz pre soaked pearl barley
- 500ml/2 cups beef stock
- 300g/11oz potatoes, peeled & diced
- Low cal cooking oil spray
- Salt & pepper to taste

## Method

**1** Preheat the oven to 160c/325f/Gas3

**2** Using a flameproof casserole dish quickly brown the beef in a little low cal oil for a few minutes. Remove the beef, add a little more oil and gently sauté the onions, celery, garlic, carrots & mushrooms for a few minutes until softened (add a splash of water if it's a little dry).

**3** Add the beef back to the casserole along with the barley, stock & potatoes. Bring to the boil, cover and place in the preheated oven to cook for approximately 2-2 ½ hours or until the beef is super tender and cooked through.

**4** Check the stew during cooking. If it needs more liquid add a little stock. If you find there is too much, remove the lid and cook for a little longer to reduce the liquid. Season and serve.

### CHEFS NOTE
Lentils make a good alternative to pearl barley in this simple one-pot dish.

# RUBY BEEF STEW

**340** calories per serving

## Ingredients

- 500g/1lb 2oz lean chuck steak, cubed
- 2 onions, chopped
- 1 celery stalk, chopped
- 1 garlic clove, crushed
- ½ turnip, chopped
- 2 large carrots, chopped
- 1 tbsp Worcestershire sauce
- 400g/14oz vine ripened tomatoes, roughly chopped
- 2 fresh beetroot bulbs, peeled & grated
- 500ml/2 cups beef stock
- Low cal cooking oil spray
- Salt & pepper to taste

## Method

**1** Preheat the oven to 160c/325f/Gas3

**2** Using a flameproof casserole dish quickly brown the beef in a little low cal oil for a few minutes. Remove the beef, add a little more oil and gently sauté the onions, celery, garlic & carrots for a few minutes until softened (add a splash of water if it's a little dry).

**3** Add the beef back to the casserole along with the Worcestershire sauce, tomatoes, grated beetroot & stock. Bring to the boil, cover and place in the preheated oven to cook for approximately 2-2 ½ hours or until the beef is super tender and cooked through.

**4** Check the stew during cooking. If it needs more liquid add a little stock. If you find there is too much, remove the lid and cook for a little longer to reduce the liquid. Season and serve.

### CHEFS NOTE

Make things easy for yourself by whizzing the beetroot in a food processor rather than grating.

# CIDER & SAGE PORK

**390**
calories per
serving

## *Ingredients*

- 600g/1lb 5oz pork tenderloin, cubed
- 2 onions, chopped
- 1 celery stalk, chopped
- 1 garlic clove, crushed
- 3 large carrots, chopped
- 2 tsp anchovy paste
- 2 apples, peeled, cored and diced
- 1 tbsp fresh sage, chopped
- 250ml/1 cup dry cider
- 250ml/1 cup chicken stock
- Low cal cooking oil spray
- Salt & pepper to taste

## *Method*

**1** Preheat the oven to 160c/325f/Gas3

**2** Using a flameproof casserole dish quickly brown the pork in a little low cal oil for a few minutes. Remove the pork, add a little more oil and gently sauté the onions, celery, garlic & carrots for a few minutes until softened (add a splash of water if it's a little dry).

**3** Add the pork back to the dish along with all the other ingredients. Bring to the boil, cover and place in the preheated oven for approximately 2 - 2 ½ hours or until the pork is tender and the apples are pulpy.

**4** Check the stew during cooking. If it needs more liquid add a little stock. If you find there is too much, remove the lid and cook for a little longer to reduce the liquid. Season and serve.

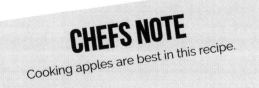

**CHEFS NOTE**
Cooking apples are best in this recipe.

# SIMPLE SPANISH PAELLA

**480**
calories per
serving

## Ingredients

- 1 onion, chopped
- 3 garlic cloves, crushed
- 50g/2oz chorizo, finely chopped
- 1 red pepper, deseeded & sliced
- 200g/7oz cherry tomatoes, halved
- 200g/7oz skinless chicken breasts, sliced
- ½ tsp cayenne pepper

- 500ml/2 cups chicken stock
- 1 tsp turmeric
- 200g/7oz paella rice
- 150g/5oz peas
- 200g/7oz raw shelled prawns, chopped
- Low cal cooking oil spray
- Salt & pepper to taste

## Method

**1** Using a heavy bottomed frying pan gently sauté the onions, garlic, chorizo, peppers & cherry tomatoes in a little low cal spray for a few minutes until softened (add a splash of water to the pan if it's a little dry). Add the chicken and cook for 2 minutes longer.

**2** Add the cayenne pepper, stock, turmeric and paella rice. Bring to the boil, cover and cook for 30 minutes.

**3** Add the peas and prawns, cover and leave to simmer for a further 8-10 minutes or until the rice is tender, the stock has been absorbed and the prawns are cooked through.

**4** Check the paella during cooking. If it needs more liquid add additional stock. Season and serve.

## CHEFS NOTE

Almost any mix of meats and seafood will work well in this versatile Spanish dish.

# SHREDDED LAMB

**495**
calories per
serving

## Ingredients

- 600g/1lb 5oz lean lamb shoulder, trimmed
- 1 tsp dried rosemary
- Pinch salt
- 3 tbsp lemon juice
- 1 tbsp each olive oil and balsamic vinegar
- 2 garlic cloves, crushed

- 1 onion, sliced
- 400g/14oz tinned chopped tomatoes
- 300g/11oz tinned flageolet beans, drained
- 120ml/½ cup chicken stock
- Salt & pepper to taste

## Method

**1** Preheat the oven to 160c/325f/Gas3

**2** Mix together the rosemary, salt, lemon juice, olive oil, balsamic vinegar & garlic. Rub this all over the lamb and season well.

**3** Sit the lamb in a flameproof casserole dish and add the onions, tomatoes, beans & stock around the sides of the lamb. Cover and place in a preheated oven for approx 2-3 hours or until the lamb is very tender.

**4** Check the stew during cooking. If it needs more liquid add a little stock.

**5** Turn the lamb half way through cooking to ensure it doesn't dry out. When the cooking time is over allow the lamb to cool for a little while and then use your hands, or two forks, to shred into thin strips.

**6** Spoon out the tomatoes and beans into shallow bowls and sit the shredded lamb on top. Check the seasoning and serve.

## CHEFS NOTE

Lamb on the bone is good for this recipe. The weight in the ingredients is for meat only. A bone-in joint will be heavier.

# BEEF & MUSTARD STEW

**439**
calories per serving

## Ingredients

- 500g/1lb 2oz lean chuck steak, cubed
- 2 garlic cloves, crushed
- 2 onions, chopped
- 2 large carrots, chopped
- 125g/4oz mushrooms, sliced
- 1 tbsp plain/all purpose flour
- 500ml/2 cups beef stock

- 1 tbsp Dijon mustard
- 1 tsp English mustard
- 1 tsp dried thyme
- 2 tsp brown sugar
- 300g/11oz potatoes, peeled & diced
- Low cal cooking oil spray
- Salt & pepper to taste

## Method

**1** Preheat the oven to 160c/325f/Gas3

**2** Using a flameproof casserole dish quickly brown the beef in a little low cal oil for a few minutes. Remove the beef, add a little more oil and gently sauté the onions, garlic, carrots & mushrooms for a few minutes until softened (add a splash of water if it's a little dry). Stir through the flour and cook for a minute or two longer.

**3** Add the stock, both mustards, sugar, thyme, potatoes and browned beef. Bring to the boil, cover and place in the preheated oven to cook for approximately 1½-2 hours, or until the beef is super tender and cooked through.

**4** Check the stew during cooking. If it needs more liquid add a little stock. If you find there is too much, remove the lid and cook for a little longer to reduce the liquid. Season and serve.

### CHEFS NOTE
Wholegrain mustard also makes a good addition to this rich stew.

# GREEK BEEF STEW

**440** calories per serving

## Ingredients

- 500g/1lb 2oz lean chuck steak, cubed
- 2 red onions, quartered
- 2 carrots, peeled & cut into batons
- 2 celery stalks, roughly sliced
- 2 tbsp freshly chopped oregano
- 400g/14oz tinned chopped tomatoes
- 2 tbsp tomato puree/paste
- ½ tsp ground cinnamon
- 2 tbsp raisins, chopped
- 1 tsp brown sugar
- Low cal cooking oil spray
- Zest of one lemon
- Salt & pepper to taste

## Method

**1** Preheat the oven to 160c/325f/Gas3

**2** Using a flameproof casserole dish quickly brown the beef in a little low cal oil for a few minutes. Remove the beef, add a little more oil and gently sauté the onions, carrots & chopped celery for a few minutes until softened (add a splash of water if it's a little dry).

**3** Add the browned beef, oregano, tomatoes, tomato puree, cinnamon, raisins & sugar.

**4** Bring to the boil, cover and place in the preheated oven to cook for approximately 1½-2 hours, or until the beef is super tender and cooked through.

**5** Check the stew during cooking. If it needs more liquid add a little stock. If you find there is too much, remove the lid and cook for a little longer to reduce the liquid. Season and serve with lemon zest sprinkled over the top of the stew.

## CHEFS NOTE

You could try orange zest as a garnish too if you wish.

# RED WINE BEEF

**460**
calories per serving

## Ingredients

- 500g/1lb 2oz lean chuck steak, cubed
- 2 onions, chopped
- 2 carrots, peeled & chopped
- 500ml/2 cups red wine
- 8 garlic cloves, peeled and left whole
- 1 tsp dried rosemary
- 1 tsp ground black pepper
- Low cal cooking oil spray
- Salt & pepper to taste

## Method

**1** Preheat the oven to 150c/300f/Gas2

**2** Using a flameproof casserole dish quickly brown the beef in a little low cal oil for a few minutes. Remove the beef, add a little more oil and gently sauté the onions & carrots for a few minutes until softened (add a splash of water if it's a little dry).

**3** Add the browned beef, red wine, garlic cloves, rosemary & black pepper. Bring to the boil, cover and place in the preheated oven to cook for approximately 2-2½ hours, or until the beef is super tender and cooked through.

**4** Check the stew during cooking. If it needs more liquid add a little stock. If you find there is too much, remove the lid and cook for a little longer to reduce the liquid. Season and serve.

## CHEFS NOTE

This tasty stew has a thin sauce which is lovely served splashed over mashed potatoes.

# BEEF & PORTABELLA STROGANOFF

**380** calories per serving

## Ingredients

- 500g/1lb 2oz lean chuck steak, cubed
- 2 onions, chopped
- 4 portabella mushrooms, thickly sliced
- 180ml/¾ cup beef stock
- 2 tbsp tomato puree/paste

- 1 tsp paprika
- 120ml/½ cup low fat crème fraiche or fat free Greek yogurt
- Low cal cooking oil spray
- Salt & pepper to taste

## Method

**1** Preheat the oven to 160c/325f/Gas3

**2** Using a flameproof casserole dish quickly brown the beef in a little low cal oil for a few minutes. Remove the beef, add a little more oil and gently sauté the onions & mushrooms for a few minutes until softened (add a splash of water if it's a little dry).

**3** Add the browned beef, stock, puree & paprika. Bring to the boil, cover and place in the preheated oven to cook for approximately 1½-2 hours, or until the beef is super tender and cooked through.

**4** Check the stew during cooking. If it needs more liquid add a little stock. If you find there is too much, remove the lid and cook for a little longer to reduce the liquid.

**5** Stir through the crème fraiche, season and serve.

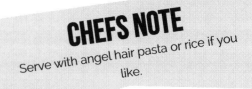

**CHEFS NOTE**
Serve with angel hair pasta or rice if you like.

# CLASSIC SHALLOT BOURGUIGNON

**460** calories per serving

## Ingredients

- 500g/1lb 2oz lean chuck steak, cubed
- 2 onions, chopped
- 2 slices lean, back bacon, chopped
- 3 garlic cloves, crushed
- 300g/11oz chestnut mushrooms, halved
- 1 tbsp plain/all purpose flour
- 1 tsp dried thyme
- 250ml/1 cup beef stock

- 120ml/½ cup red wine
- 20g/1oz low fat 'butter' spread
- 10 shallots, peeled & halved
- Low cal cooking oil spray
- Handful of freshly chopped flat leaf parsley
- Salt & pepper to taste

## Method

**1** Preheat the oven to 160c/325f/Gas3

**2** Using a flameproof casserole dish quickly brown the beef in a little low cal oil for a few minutes. Remove the beef, add a little more oil and gently sauté the onions, bacon, garlic & mushrooms for a few minutes until softened (add a splash of water if it's a little dry).

**3** Place the beef in a plastic bag with the flour and shake until the beef is lightly covered in all the flour.

**4** Add the floured beef, thyme, stock & wine. Bring to the boil, cover and place in the preheated oven to cook for approximately 1½-2 hours, or until the beef is super tender and cooked through.

**5** Check the stew during cooking. If it needs more liquid add a little stock. If you find there is too much, remove the lid and cook for a little longer to reduce the liquid.

**6** As the stew nears the end of it's cooking time gently sauté the shallots in a frying pan with the 'butter' for at least 10 minutes on a very gentle heat to caramelise.

**7** When the stew is ready stir through the shallots, check the seasoning and serve with chopped parsley.

# SMOKED HAM & CREAM CHEESE RISOTTO

**450** calories per serving

## Ingredients

- 1 tbsp olive oil
- 1 onion, chopped
- 1 leek, sliced
- 1 garlic clove, crushed
- 250g/9oz risotto rice

- 125g/4oz smoked ham, chopped
- 200g/7oz peas
- 750g/3 cups vegetable stock
- 3 tbsp low fat cream cheese
- Salt & pepper to taste

## Method

**1** Preheat the oven to 180c/350f/Gas4

**2** Using a flameproof casserole dish gently sauté the onion, leek & garlic in the olive oil for about 5 minutes until softened.

**3** Add the rice and stir well for a minute or two until every grain of rice is coated with the olive oil.

**4** Add the ham, peas & stock and bring to the boil. Cover and place in the preheated oven for 25-30 minutes or until the risotto is tender and the stock has been absorbed.

**5** Check the risotto during cooking. If it needs more liquid add a little stock. If you find there is too much, remove the lid and cook for a little longer to reduce the stock.

**6** Remove from the oven, stir through the cream cheese, season & serve.

### CHEFS NOTE
You could use gammon or bacon instead of smoked ham if you wish.

# SAUSAGE GOULASH

**430** calories per serving

## Ingredients

- 8 lean pork sausages
- 2 onions, chopped
- 2 garlic cloves, crushed
- 1 red pepper, deseeded & sliced
- 200g/7oz chestnut mushrooms, halved
- 1 tsp paprika
- ½ tsp cayenne pepper or chilli powder
- 1 tbsp plain/all purpose flour

- 400g/14oz tinned chopped tomatoes
- 250ml/1 cup beef stock
- 4 tbsp fat free Greek yogurt
- Low cal cooking oil spray
- Handful of freshly chopped flat leaf parsley
- Salt & pepper to taste

## Method

**1** Preheat the oven to 160c/325f/Gas3

**2** Using a flameproof casserole dish quickly brown the sausages in a little low cal oil for a few minutes. Remove the sausages and slice into 1cm/½ inch thick rounds.

**3** Add a little more oil to the casserole and gently sauté the onions, garlic, peppers & mushrooms for a few minutes until softened (add a splash of water if it's a little dry). Stir through the flour, paprika & cayenne pepper and cook for a minute or two longer. Add the sliced sausages, tomatoes & stock.

**4** Quickly bring to the boil, cover and place in the preheated oven to cook for approximately 1-1½ hours, or until the stew is thick and piping hot.

**5** Check the stew during cooking. If it needs more liquid add a little stock. If you find there is too much, remove the lid and cook for a little longer to reduce the liquid.

**6** Season and serve with a tablespoon of fat free Greek yogurt on top sprinkled with chopped parsley.

## CHEFS NOTE

Increase the cayenne pepper if you prefer your goulash to have a 'kick'.

# BEEF COCONUT STEW

475
calories per
serving

## Ingredients

- 600g/1lb 5oz lean chuck steak, cubed
- 1 onion, sliced
- 1 green pepper, deseeded & sliced
- 1 tbsp freshly grated ginger
- 2 carrots, peeled & cut into batons
- 1 red chilli, deseeded & finely sliced
- 3 tbsp Thai fish sauce

- 1 tsp brown sugar
- 400g/14oz tinned chopped tomatoes
- 120ml/½ cup beef stock
- 250ml/1 cup low fat coconut milk
- Lime wedges to serve
- Low cal cooking oil spray
- Salt & pepper to taste

## Method

1 Using a flameproof casserole dish quickly brown the beef in a little low cal oil for a couple of minutes.

2 Remove the beef, add a little more oil and gently sauté the onions, peppers, ginger, carrots & chilli for a few minutes until softened (add a splash of water if it's a little dry). Add the fish sauce, sugar, chopped tomatoes & stock. Bring to the boil, cover and leave to gently simmer for an hour. Stir through the coconut milk and continue to gently simmer for a few minutes until the beef is tender and the stew is piping hot.

3 Check the stew during cooking. If it needs more liquid add a little stock. If you find there is too much, remove the lid and cook for a little longer to reduce the liquid. Season and serve with lime wedges

## CHEFS NOTE

Try serving with some chopped peanuts and boiled rice.

# LAMB & LENTILS

**460** calories per serving

## Ingredients

- 125g/3oz red lentils
- 500g/1lb 2oz lean lamb shoulder, cubed
- 2 onions, sliced
- 3 garlic cloves, crushed
- 400g/14oz tinned chopped tomatoes
- 1 tbsp curry powder
- 120ml/½ cup chicken stock
- 125g/4oz baby corn, sliced lengthways
- Small bunch freshly chopped coriander/cilantro
- Low cal cooking oil spray
- Salt & pepper to taste

## Method

**1** Soak the lentils in cold water for an hour.

**2** Using a flameproof casserole dish quickly brown the lamb in a little low cal oil for a couple of minutes. Remove the lamb, add a little more oil and gently sauté the onions & garlic for a few minutes until softened (add a splash of water if it's a little dry).

**3** Add the tomatoes, curry powder, stock & pre-soaked lentils. Bring to the boil, cover and leave to gently simmer for at least an hour or until the lamb is tender and the lentils are cooked through. Add the baby corn 5-10 minutes before the end of cooking time.

**4** Check the stew during cooking. If it needs more liquid add a little stock. If you find there is too much, remove the lid and cook for a little longer to reduce the liquid. Season and serve with freshly chopped coriander.

## CHEFS NOTE

Green lentils or yellow split peas will also work well in this stew.

# MOROCCAN LAMB & ONIONS

**440** calories per serving

## Ingredients

- 500g/1lb 2oz lean lamb shoulder, cubed
- 3 onions, sliced
- 1 tsp brown sugar
- 3 garlic cloves, crushed
- 400g/14oz vine ripened tomatoes, roughly chopped
- 2 tbsp tomato puree/paste
- 1 tbsp honey
- 1 tsp each ground coriander/cilantro & turmeric
- ½ tsp each ground cinnamon & allspice
- 50g/2oz dried apricots, chopped
- 1 large sweet potato, peeled & diced
- 2 tbsp raisins, chopped
- 120ml/½ cup chicken stock
- Low cal cooking oil spray
- Salt & pepper to taste

## Method

**1** Using a flameproof casserole dish quickly brown the lamb in a little low cal oil for a couple of minutes. Remove the lamb, add a little more oil and gently sauté the onions, sugar & garlic for about 10 minutes until very soft (add a splash of water if it's a little dry).

**2** Add the tomatoes, puree, honey, dried spices, apricots, sweet potato, raisins & stock. Bring to the boil, cover and leave to gently simmer for 1-1 ½ hours or until the lamb is very tender.

**3** Check the stew during cooking. If it needs more liquid add a little stock. If you find there is too much, remove the lid and cook for a little longer to reduce the liquid. Season and serve.

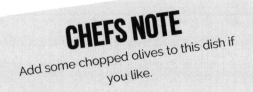

**CHEFS NOTE**
Add some chopped olives to this dish if you like.

# SWEET BEEF

**460**
calories per
serving

## Ingredients

- 1 tbsp plain/all purpose flour
- 500g/1lb 2oz lean chuck steak, cubed
- 2 onions, sliced
- 2 garlic cloves, crushed
- 2 parsnips, peeled & chopped
- 2 carrots, peeled & chopped
- 2 tsp honey
- 500ml/2 cups beef stock
- 1 butternut squash, peeled, deseeded & cubed
- Low cal cooking oil spray
- Salt & pepper to taste

## Method

**1** Dust the beef with flour. Using a flameproof casserole dish quickly brown the floured beef in a little low cal oil for a couple of minutes. Remove the beef, add a little more oil and gently sauté the onions, garlic, parsnips & carrots for a few minutes until softened (add a splash of water if it's a little dry).

**2** Add the honey, stock & squash. Bring to the boil, cover and leave to gently simmer for 1½-2 hours or until the beef is very tender and the stew is piping hot.

**3** Check the stew during cooking. If it needs more liquid add a little stock. If you find there is too much, remove the lid and cook for a little longer to reduce the liquid. Season and serve.

## CHEFS NOTE
Place the flour and steak in a plastic bag and shake to evenly cover the beef.

# SPICED PORK & BUTTER-BEAN STEW

**380** calories per serving

## Ingredients

- 500g/1lb 2oz pork tenderloin, cubed
- 1 onion, chopped
- 1 red chilli, deseeded & finely chopped
- 2 garlic cloves, crushed
- 3 slices lean, back bacon, chopped
- 400g/14oz tinned butter beans, drained
- 400g/14oz vine ripened tomatoes, chopped
- 1 tsp brown sugar
- 60ml/¼ cup chicken stock
- Low cal cooking oil spray
- Salt & pepper to taste

## Method

**1** Using a flameproof casserole dish quickly brown the pork in a little low cal oil for a couple of minutes. Remove the pork, add a little more oil and gently sauté the onions, chilli, garlic & chopped bacon for a few minutes until softened.

**2** Add all the ingredients to the casserole dish, combine well and bring to a simmer. Cover and cook for 45–60 mins or until the stew is bubbling hot and cooked through.

**3** Check often during cooking. If it needs more liquid add a little stock. If you find there is too much, remove the lid and cook for a little longer to reduce the liquid. Season and serve.

**CHEFS NOTE**
Borlotti or flageolet beans will also work well in this stew.

# PILAF ONE-POT

**350** calories per serving

## Ingredients

- 1 onion, chopped
- 2 garlic cloves, crushed
- ½ tsp ground cumin, turmeric & chilli powder
- 200g/7oz lean minced/ground beef

- 200g/7oz long grain rice
- 150g/5oz green beans, chopped
- 750ml/3 cups beef stock
- Low cal cooking oil spray
- Salt & pepper to taste

## Method

**1** Using a flameproof casserole dish gently sauté the onions & garlic in a little low cal spray for a few minutes until the onions are softened (add a splash of water if it's a little dry).

**2** Add the dried spices & beef and cook for a few minutes. Add the rice, beans & stock. Cover and gently simmer for 15-20 minutes or until the rice is cooked through and the stock is absorbed.

**3** Check the pilaf during cooking. If it needs more liquid add a little stock. If you find there is too much, remove the lid and cook for a little longer to reduce the liquid. Season and serve.

### CHEFS NOTE
Chopped coriander/cilantro makes a good garnish for this dish.

# Skinny
# ONE POT
# POULTRY
## DISHES

# CHICKEN & CHORIZO RICE STEW

**490** calories per serving

## Ingredients

- 1 onion, chopped
- 2 garlic cloves, crushed
- 100g/3½oz chorizo, sliced & chopped
- 1 red pepper, deseeded & sliced
- 1 red chilli, deseeded & finely chopped
- 4 skinless chicken breasts, each weighing 125g/4oz
- 200g/7oz tinned chopped tomatoes
- 500ml/2 cups chicken stock
- 200g/7oz long grain rice
- 2 tbsp tomato puree/paste
- 2 bay leaves
- Lemon wedges to serve
- Low cal cooking oil spray
- Salt & pepper to taste

## Method

**1** Using a flameproof casserole dish gently sauté the onions, garlic, chorizo, pepper & chopped chillies in a little low cal spray for a few minutes until softened (add a splash of water if it's a little dry). Remove to a plate, add a little more oil to the casserole dish, increase the heat and quickly brown the chicken breasts for a few minutes.

**2** Add all the ingredients back into the casserole dish and combine well. Bring to a hard simmer, cover, reduce the heat and leave to gently cook for 20-25 minutes or until the rice is tender and the chicken is cooked through.

**3** Check the stew during cooking. If it needs more liquid add a little stock. If you find there is too much, remove the lid and cook for a little longer to reduce the liquid.

**4** Remove the bay leaves, check the seasoning and serve with lemon wedges.

## CHEFS NOTE

Try shredding the chicken breasts after cooking and stir back through the stew.

# COCONUT MILK & CHICKEN LIGHT STEW

**295** calories per serving

## Ingredients

- 1 onion, chopped
- 2 garlic cloves, crushed
- 1 red chilli, deseeded & finely chopped
- 400g/14oz skinless chicken breast, cubed
- 125g/4oz baby corn, sliced lengthways
- 125g/4oz peas
- 200g/7oz cherry tomatoes, halved
- 2 tbsp tomato puree/paste
- 120ml/½ cup low fat coconut milk
- Small bunch fresh coriander/cilantro, roughly chopped
- Lime wedges to serve
- Low cal cooking oil spray
- Salt & pepper to taste

## Method

**1** Using a flameproof casserole dish gently sauté the onions, garlic & chopped chillies in a little low cal spray for a few minutes until softened (add a splash of water if it's a little dry). Remove to a plate, add a little more oil to the casserole dish, increase the heat and quickly brown the chicken for a few minutes.

**2** Add all the sautéed vegetables, baby corn, peas, cherry tomatoes & puree back into the casserole dish and combine well. Gently cook for 5 minutes. Add the coconut milk & chopped coriander, cover and leave to gently cook for 20-25 minutes or until the stew is piping hot and the chicken is cooked through.

**3** Check the stew during cooking. If it needs more liquid add a little stock. If you find there is too much, remove the lid and cook for a little longer to reduce the liquid.

**4** Check the seasoning and serve with lime wedges.

### CHEFS NOTE
Reserve a little of the chopped coriander to use as a garnish.

# CHICKEN & ROSEMARY

**298** calories per serving

## Ingredients

- 1 onion, chopped
- 1 leek, chopped
- 1 celery stalk, chopped
- 2 large carrots, chopped
- 2 garlic cloves, crushed
- 4 skinless chicken breasts, each weighing 125g/4oz
- 1 tbsp plain/all purpose flour
- 500g/2 cups chicken stock
- 1 tbsp Dijon mustard
- Small bunch fresh rosemary, roughly chopped
- 200g/7oz green beans
- 2 handfuls shredded cabbage or spring greens
- Low cal cooking oil spray
- Salt & pepper to taste

## Method

**1** Using a flameproof casserole dish quickly brown the chicken breasts in a little low cal oil for a couple of minutes. Remove the chicken, add a little more oil and gently sauté the onions, leek, celery, carrots & garlic for a few minutes until softened (add a splash of water if it's a little dry). Stir through the flour until well combined.

**2** Add the stock & mustard and cook for two minutes stirring throughout. Add the rosemary, cover and leave to gently cook for 40-50 minutes or until the stew is piping hot and the chicken is cooked through.

**3** Five minutes before the end of cooking add the green beans and cabbage (add earlier if you prefer them tender).

**4** Check the stew during cooking. If it needs more liquid add a little stock. If you find there is too much, remove the lid and cook for a little longer to reduce the liquid.

**5** Check the seasoning and serve.

## CHEFS NOTE

A tablespoon of fat free Greek yogurt makes a good addition to this stew when serving.

# CHICKEN & WHITE WINE CASSEROLE

**340** calories per serving

## Ingredients

- 4 skinless chicken breasts, each weighing 150g/5oz
- 2 onions, chopped
- 4 garlic cloves, crushed
- 3 large carrots, chopped
- 200g/7oz mushrooms, sliced
- 250ml/1 cup dry white wine
- 120ml/½ cup chicken stock
- Lemon wedges to serve
- Low cal cooking oil spray
- Salt & pepper to taste

## Method

**1** Using a flameproof casserole dish quickly brown the chicken in a little low cal oil for a few minutes. Remove the chicken to a plate, add a little more oil and gently sauté the onions, garlic, carrots & mushrooms for a few minutes until softened (add a splash of water if it's a little dry).

**2** Add the chicken and wine to the casserole and bring to the boil for 2 minutes. Add the stock, cover and gently simmer for 20-30 minutes or until the chicken is cooked through.

**3** Check the stew during cooking. If it needs more liquid add a little stock. If you find there is too much, remove the lid and cook for a little longer to reduce the liquid. Season and serve.

### CHEFS NOTE
This stew is great served with mashed potatoes and chopped flat leaf parsley.

# FRESH TOMATO & BASIL ONE-POT CHICKEN

**345** calories per serving

## Ingredients

- 2 onions, chopped
- 6 garlic cloves, crushed
- 600g/1lb 5oz vine ripened tomatoes, roughly chopped
- 4 skinless chicken breasts, each weighing 150g/5oz
- 120ml/½ cup red wine
- 120ml/½ cup chicken stock
- Large bunch fresh basil, chopped
- 1 bay leaf
- Low cal cooking oil spray
- Salt & pepper to taste

## Method

1 Using a flameproof casserole dish, gently sauté the onions, garlic & tomatoes for a few minutes until softened.

2 Add the chicken, wine, basil & bay leaf and bring to the boil for 2 minutes. Add the stock, cover and gently simmer for 30-40 minutes or until the chicken is cooked through and tender.

3 Check the stew during cooking. If it needs more liquid add a little stock. If you find there is too much, remove the lid and cook for a little longer to reduce the liquid. Season and serve.

**CHEFS NOTE**
Reserve a little of the basil as a garnish.

# AROMATIC CHICKEN STEW

**490** calories per serving

## Ingredients

- 400g/14oz skinless chicken breasts, cubed
- 2 onions, sliced
- 3 garlic cloves, crushed
- 200g/7oz tinned chickpeas, drained
- 1 tsp each turmeric & cumin
- ½ tsp each ground cinnamon & cardamom
- 750ml/3 cups chicken stock
- 200g/7oz brown rice
- 2 tbsp chopped raisins
- Low cal cooking oil spray
- Salt & pepper to taste

## Method

**1** Preheat the oven to 180c/350f/Gas4

**2** Using a flameproof casserole dish gently sauté the onions & garlic in a little low cal spray for a few minutes until softened.

**3** Add all the ingredients to the casserole, combine well and bring to the boil. Cover the casserole dish, transfer to the preheated oven and cook for 1-1 ½ hours or until the rice is tender, the stock has been absorbed and the chicken is cooked through.

**4** Check the stew during cooking. If it needs more liquid add a little stock. If you find there is too much, remove the lid and cook for a little longer to reduce the liquid. Season and serve.

### CHEFS NOTE
Brown rice is a great choice as it retains a firm texture but feel free to use white rice if you prefer.

# SPICED CHICKEN & OLIVES

**460** calories per serving

## Ingredients

- 500g/1lb 2oz skinless chicken breasts, cubed
- 2 onions, sliced
- 3 garlic cloves, crushed
- 2 green chillies, deseeded & finely chopped
- 1 tsp turmeric
- ½ tsp cayenne pepper
- 200g/7oz tinned Borlotti beans, drained
- 50g/2oz black, pitted olives, halved
- 400g/14oz tinned chopped tomatoes
- 120ml/½ cup chicken stock
- 2 tbsp fat free Greek yogurt
- Low cal cooking oil spray
- Salt & pepper to taste

## Method

**1** Using a flameproof casserole dish quickly brown the chicken in a little low cal oil for a couple of minutes. Remove the chicken to a plate, add a little more oil and gently sauté the onions, garlic & chilli for a few minutes until softened (add a splash of water if it's a little dry).

**2** Add the turmeric, cayenne pepper, beans, olives, tomatoes & stock. Bring to the boil, cover and leave to gently simmer cook for 30 minutes or until the chicken is tender.

**3** Check the stew during cooking. If it needs more liquid add a little stock. If you find there is too much, remove the lid and cook for a little longer to reduce the liquid.

**4** Stir through the yogurt until gently warmed, season and serve.

### CHEFS NOTE
Use pitted Kalamata olives if you can get them.

# HONEY MUSTARD CHICKEN

**320**
calories per serving

## Ingredients

- 4 chicken breasts, each weighing 5oz/150g
- 2 onions, sliced
- 1 red pepper, deseeded & sliced
- 2 garlic cloves, crushed
- 4 carrots, peeled & sliced into batons
- 1 tbsp honey
- 250ml/1 cup chicken stock
- 1 tsp dried thyme
- Low cal cooking oil spray
- Salt & pepper to taste

## Method

1 Using a flameproof casserole dish quickly brown the chicken in a little low cal oil for a couple of minutes. Remove the chicken, add a little more oil and gently sauté the onions, peppers, garlic & carrots for a few minutes until softened (add a splash of water if it's a little dry).

2 Add the honey, stock and thyme. Bring to the boil, cover and leave to gently simmer for about 40 mins or until the carrots are tender and the chicken is cooked through.

3 Check during cooking. If it needs more liquid add a little stock. If you find there is too much, remove the lid and cook for a little longer to reduce the liquid. Season and serve.

**CHEFS NOTE**
This is great served with a mound of steamed savoy cabbage.

# AFRICAN CHICKEN ONE-POT

**495** calories per serving

## Ingredients

- 500g/1lb 2oz skinless chicken breasts, cubed
- 1 red onion, sliced
- 3 garlic cloves, crushed
- 2 tsp freshly grated ginger
- 2 red chillies, deseeded & finely chopped
- 400g/14oz tinned chopped tomatoes
- 100g/3½oz low fat peanut butter
- 120ml/½ cup chicken stock
- 300g/11oz sweet potatoes, peeled & cubed
- 100g/3½oz peas
- 125g/4oz watercress
- Low cal cooking oil spray
- Salt & pepper to taste

## Method

**1** Using a flameproof casserole dish quickly brown the chicken in a little low cal oil for a couple of minutes. Remove the chicken, add a little more oil and gently sauté the onions, garlic, ginger & chillies for a few minutes until softened (add a splash of wate if it's a little dry).

**2** Add the tomatoes, peanut butter, stock, sweet potatoes & peas. Bring to the boil, cover and leave to gently simmer cook for 30 minutes or until the chicken is tender.

**3** Check the stew during cooking. If it needs more liquid add a little stock. If you find there is too much, remove the lid and cook for a little longer to reduce the liquid. Season and serve with a pile of fresh watercress.

### CHEFS NOTE
Use smooth or crunchy peanut butter, either will work well.

# LENTIL CHICKEN CASSEROLE

**380** calories per serving

## Ingredients

- 3 slices lean, back bacon, chopped
- 500g/1lb 2oz chicken breasts, chopped
- 1 onion, sliced
- 1 red pepper, deseeded & sliced
- 1 garlic clove, crushed
- 2 tbsp tomato puree/paste
- 500ml/2 cups chicken stock
- 125g/4oz lentils
- 1 tsp dried thyme
- Low cal cooking oil spray
- Salt & pepper to taste

## Method

**1** Using a flameproof casserole dish quickly brown the bacon and chicken in a little low cal oil for a couple of minutes. Remove the bacon and chicken to a plate, add a little more oil and gently sauté the onions, peppers & garlic for a few minutes until softened (add a splash of water if it's a little dry).

**2** Add the puree, stock, lentils and thyme. Bring to the boil, cover and leave to gently simmer for about 40 mins or until the lentils are tender and the stock has reduced.

**3** Check the casserole during cooking. If it needs more liquid add a little stock. If you find there is too much, remove the lid and cook for a little longer to reduce the liquid. Season and serve.

### CHEFS NOTE
A handful of mushrooms or green beans makes a good addition to this casserole.

# Skinny
# ONE POT
# VEGETABLE
## DISHES

# MIXED BEAN TAGINE

**360**
calories per serving

## Ingredients

- 1 onion, chopped
- 2 garlic cloves, crushed
- 1 red pepper, deseeded & sliced
- 1 aubergine/egg plant, cubed
- 1 red chilli, deseeded & finely chopped
- 3 large vine ripened tomatoes, chopped
- 1 tsp ground paprika

- 2 tbsp tomato puree/paste
- 250ml/1 cup vegetable stock
- ½ tsp ground coriander/cilantro
- 800g/1¾lb tinned mixed beans, drained
- 4 tbsp fat free Greek yogurt
- Low cal cooking oil spray
- Salt & pepper to taste

## Method

**1** Using a flameproof casserole dish gently sauté the onions, garlic, peppers, aubergine, chillies & tomatoes in little low cal spray for about 10 minutes until softened (add a splash of water if it's a little dry).

**2** Add the paprika, puree, stock & coriander. Cover and gently simmer for 10 minutes.

**3** Add the mixed beans and cook for a further 20 minutes or until everything is tender and piping hot.

**4** Check the beans during cooking. If they need more liquid add a little stock. If you find there is too much, remove the lid and cook for a little longer to reduce the liquid.

**5** Season and serve with a dollop of fat free Greek yogurt on top.

### CHEFS NOTE
Freshly chopped mint mixed through the Greek yogurt makes a good addition.

# AROMATIC CHICKPEA & GREENS

**295** calories per serving

## Ingredients

- 1 onion, chopped
- 2 garlic cloves, crushed
- 1 red pepper, deseeded & sliced
- 1 green chilli, deseeded & finely chopped
- 1 tbsp curry powder
- 1 tsp each turmeric & cumin
- 400g/14oz tinned, chopped tomatoes
- 250ml/1 cup vegetable stock
- 2 tbsp tomato puree/paste
- 800g/1¾lb tinned chickpeas, drained
- 200g/7oz spinach leaves
- Low cal cooking oil spray
- Salt & pepper to taste

## Method

**1** Preheat the oven to 180c/350f/Gas4

**2** Using a flameproof casserole dish gently sauté the onions, garlic, peppers & chill in a little low cal spray for a few minutes until softened (add a splash of water if it's a little dry).

**3** Add the curry powder, turmeric, cumin, chopped tomatoes, stock, puree & chickpeas. Combine well and bring to the boil. Cover the casserole dish, transfer to the preheated oven and cook for 1-1 ½ hours or until the stew is bubbling hot and cooked through.

**4** Check the stew during cooking. If it needs more liquid add a little stock. If you find there is too much, remove the lid and cook for a little longer to reduce the liquid.

**5** Stir through the spinach leaves, check the seasoning and serve.

### CHEFS NOTE
Adding the spinach at the end of the cooking time will give the stew a fresh 'crunch'.

# CREAMY BUTTERNUT SQUASH STEW

**400** calories per serving

## Ingredients

- 2 butternut squash, peeled & deseeded
- 2 onions, chopped
- 2 garlic cloves, crushed
- 2 carrots, thickly sliced
- 1 tsp dried rosemary
- 250g/9oz lentils
- 1lt/4 cups vegetable stock
- 60ml/¼ cup low fat cream
- Low cal cooking oil spray
- Salt & pepper to taste

## Method

**1** Cut the squash into chunks.

**2** Using a flameproof casserole dish gently sauté the onions, garlic, carrots & rosemary in little low cal spray for about 10 minutes until softened (add a splash of water if it's a little dry).

**3** Add the lentils, stock & squash chunks. Cover and gently simmer for 40-50 minutes or until the lentils are tender and the squash is cooked through.

**4** Check during cooking. If it needs more liquid add a little stock. If you find there is too much, remove the lid and cook for a little longer to reduce the liquid.

**5** Remove a ladle of the stew and blitz in a food processor until smooth (this will create a thicker, creamier texture to the stew). Return to the stew, stir through the cream and serve.

**CHEFS NOTE**

This is a super creamy stew, which is lovely served with salad or bread.

# CINNAMON LENTILS

**480** calories per serving

## Ingredients

- 1 onion, chopped
- 2 garlic cloves, crushed
- 2 carrots, chopped
- 1 parsnip, chopped
- 1 tsp dried mixed herbs
- 400g/14oz lentils
- 1.25lt/5 cups vegetable stock

- 1 tsp ground cinnamon
- 1 red onion, sliced
- 200g/7oz cherry tomatoes, halved
- 1 tbsp olive oil
- Low cal cooking oil spray
- Salt & pepper to taste

## Method

**1** Using a flameproof casserole dish gently sauté the onions, garlic, carrots, parsnip & dried herbs in little low cal spray for a few minutes until softened (add a splash of water if it's a little dry).

**2** Add the lentils, stock & cinnamon. Cover and gently simmer for 40-50 minutes or until the lentils are tender.

**3** Check the lentils during cooking. If they need more liquid add a little stock. If you find there is too much, remove the lid and cook for a little longer to reduce the liquid.

**4** Combine the tomatoes, sliced red onion & olive oil together with a little salt and pepper. Serve the lentils in shallow bowls with the onion mix piled on top.

### CHEFS NOTE
Use red or green lentils in this simple dish.

51

# SHALLOT & PEA ONE-POT RISOTTO

**390** calories per serving

## Ingredients

- 1 tbsp olive oil
- 12 shallots, chopped
- 1 leek, sliced
- 1 garlic clove, crushed
- 250g/9oz risotto rice
- 200g/7oz peas
- 750g/3 cups vegetable stock
- 2 tbsp low fat cream cheese
- Salt & pepper to taste

## Method

**1** Preheat the oven to 180c/350f/Gas4

**2** Using a flameproof casserole dish gently sauté the shallots, leeks & garlic in the olive oil for about 5 minutes until softened.

**3** Add the rice and stir well for a minute or two until every grain of rice is coated with the olive oil.

**4** Add the stock & peas and bring to the boil. Cover and place in the preheated oven for 25-30 minutes or until the risotto is tender and the stock has been absorbed.

**5** Check the risotto during cooking. If it needs more liquid add a little stock. If you find there is too much, remove the lid and cook for a little longer to reduce the stock.

**6** Remove from the oven, stir through the cream cheese, season & serve.

## CHEFS NOTE

Try adding some Parmesan cheese or chopped basil to this simple risotto.

# COURGETTE & FLAGEOLET STEW

**290**
calories per serving

## Ingredients

- 2 onions, chopped
- 2 garlic cloves, crushed
- 300g/11oz courgettes/zucchini, sliced into batons
- 2 tbsp tomato puree/paste
- 400g/14oz tinned chopped tomatoes
- 120ml/½ cup vegetable stock
- 400g/14oz tinned flageolet beans
- 200g/7oz peas
- Zest of one lemon
- Bunch freshly chopped basil
- Low cal cooking oil spray
- Salt & pepper to taste

## Method

**1** Using a flameproof casserole dish, gently sauté the onions, garlic & courgettes in little low cal spray for a few minutes until softened (add a splash of water if it's a little dry).

**2** Add the puree, chopped tomatoes & stock. Cover and gently simmer for 30 minutes or until the lentils are tender. Add the beans, peas and lemon zest. Stir and leave to cook for a further 10 minutes or until everything is tender and piping hot.

**3** Check often during cooking. If it needs more liquid add a little stock. If you find there is too much, remove the lid and cook for a little longer to reduce the liquid.

**4** Season and serve with chopped basil.

### CHEFS NOTE
Dried beans are fine to use too, provided they are soaked overnight.

# SWEETCORN & BROAD BEAN CASSEROLE

**340** calories per serving

## Ingredients

- 1 red onion, chopped
- 2 garlic cloves, crushed
- 1 red pepper, deseeded & finely chopped
- 300g/11oz sweetcorn
- 400g/14oz tinned broad beans, drained
- 2 large sweet potatoes, peeled & cubed
- 4 tbsp low fat crème fraiche or sour cream
- Low cal cooking oil spray
- Salt & pepper to taste

## Method

1 Using a flameproof casserole dish, gently sauté the onions, garlic & peppers in little low cal spray for a few minutes until softened (add a splash of water if it's a little dry).

2 Add the sweetcorn, broad beans & sweet potatoes and gently simmer for 15-20 minutes or until the sweet potatoes are tender.

3 Check the casserole during cooking. If it needs more liquid add a little stock. If you find there is too much, increase the heat to reduce the liquid.

4 Stir through the crème fraiche, season and serve.

**CHEFS NOTE**
Try adding some slices of raw red onion and chopped parsley when serving.

# STILTON PUY STEW

**290**
calories per
serving

## Ingredients

- 1 onion, sliced
- 2 celery stalks, chopped
- 2 garlic cloves, crushed
- 200g/7oz mushrooms, sliced
- 120ml/½ cup white wine
- 300g/11oz puy lentils
- 1 tsp ground cumin

- 1lt/4 cups vegetable stock
- 1 beetroot bulb, grated
- Large bunch spring onions/scallions finely chopped
- Low cal cooking oil spray
- Salt & pepper to taste

## Method

**1** Preheat the oven to 160c/325f/Gas3

**2** Gently sauté the onions, celery, garlic & mushrooms for a few minutes until softened (add a splash of water if it's a little dry). Add the white wine and increase the heat. Simmer for 3-4 minutes until the liquid has reduced by half.

**3** Add the lentils, cumin & stock. Bring to the boil, cover and place in the preheated oven to cook for 40 minutes or until the lentils are tender.

**4** Check the stew during cooking. If it needs more liquid add a little stock. If you find there is too much, remove the lid and cook for a little longer to reduce the liquid.

**5** Season and serve in shallow bowls with grated beetroot and spring onions sprinkled over the top.

### CHEFS NOTE
A little crumbled feta cheese makes a lovely additional garnish.

# GOATS CHEESE & MUSHROOMS

**280**
calories per
serving

## Ingredients

- 50g/2oz porcini mushrooms
- 2 onions, sliced
- 2 garlic cloves, crushed
- 800g/1¾lb mixed mushrooms
- 2 tbsp tomato puree/paste

- 120ml/½ cup red wine
- 1 tsp dried thyme
- 125g/4oz low fat feta cheese, crumbled
- Low cal cooking oil spray
- Salt & pepper to taste

## Method

**1** Soak the porcini mushrooms in a little warm water for 10 minutes until rehydrated. Drain and finely chop.

**2** Using a flameproof casserole dish, gently sauté the onions, garlic, porcini mushrooms & mixed mushrooms in little low cal spray for 10-15 minutes or until softened (add a splash of water if it's a little dry).

**3** Stir through the tomato puree then add the wine and thyme. Bring to the boil, reduce the heat and simmer for 5-10 minutes or until the liquid has reduced by half.

**4** Check during cooking. If it needs more liquid add a little stock. If you find there is too much, increase the heat to reduce the liquid.

**5** Stir through the crumbled feta cheese, season and serve.

### CHEFS NOTE
This is lovely served on bruschetta or toasted brown bread.

# CALABRIAN STEW

**290** calories per serving

## Ingredients

- 1 tbsp olive oil
- 2 aubergine/egg plant, cubed
- 2 onions, sliced
- 4 garlic cloves, crushed
- 800g/1¾lb tinned chopped tomatoes
- 1 tsp brown sugar
- 150g/5oz pitted olives, sliced
- 1 tbsp capers, chopped
- 2 tbsp raisins, chopped
- 2 tbsp tomato puree/paste
- 2 tbsp balsamic vinegar
- 2 tbsp pine nuts
- Low cal cooking oil spray
- Salt & pepper to taste

## Method

**1** Using a flameproof casserole dish, gently sauté the aubergine, onions & garlic in the olive oil for 10-15 minutes or until softened (add a splash of water if it's a little dry).

**2** Add the chopped tomatoes, sugar, olives, capers, raisins, puree & vinegar. Bring to the boil, reduce the heat and simmer for 20-30 minutes or until the liquid has reduced by half.

**3** Check often during cooking. If it needs more liquid add a little stock. If you find there is too much, increase the heat to reduce the liquid.

**4** Meanwhile gently brown the pine nuts in a dry pan for a minute or two (don't let them burn.). Season the stew and serve with the pine nuts sprinkled over the top.

## CHEFS NOTE

This southern Italian stew is also good served with fresh basil or a dollop of green pesto.

# SWEET POTATO & GREEN BEAN DHAL

**420** calories per serving

## Ingredients

- 1 onion, sliced
- 1 green chilli, deseeded & finely sliced
- 1 tsp freshly grated ginger
- 2 celery stalks, chopped
- 2 garlic cloves, crushed
- 1 tbsp curry powder
- 1 tsp paprika
- 400g/14oz tinned chopped tomatoes

- 250g/9oz precooked yellow split peas
- 600g/1lb 5oz sweet potato, peeled & diced
- 1 vegetable stock cube, crumbled
- 250g/9oz green beans
- 2 tbsp lemon juice
- Low cal cooking oil spray
- Salt & pepper to taste

## Method

**1** Gently sauté the onions, chilli, ginger, celery & garlic for a few minutes until softened (add a splash of water to the pan if it's a little dry).

**2** Add the curry powder, paprika, chopped tomatoes, split peas, sweet potatoes & crumbled stock cube. Cover and gently simmer for 20 minutes.

**3** Add the green beans and cook for 5 minutes longer or until the beans and sweet potatoes are tender.

**4** Check the stew during cooking. If it needs more liquid add a little stock. If you find there is too much, remove the lid and cook for a little longer to reduce the liquid.

**5** Season, stir through the lemon juice & serve.

### CHEFS NOTE
Add a little freshly chopped coriander if you have any to hand.

# OVEN BAKED PORCINI & TOMATO RISOTTO

**350** calories per serving

## Ingredients

- 50g/2oz porcini mushrooms
- 1 tbsp olive oil
- 1 onion, chopped
- 1 leek, sliced
- 1 garlic clove, crushed
- 250g/9oz cherry tomatoes, halved
- 250g/9oz risotto rice
- 750g/3 cups vegetable stock
- Bunch fresh basil, chopped
- Salt & pepper to taste

## Method

**1** Preheat the oven to 180c/350f/Gas4

**2** Soak the porcini mushrooms is a little warm water and leave to rehydrate for 10 minutes. Drain and finely chop.

**3** Using a flameproof casserole dish gently sauté the onion, leek, garlic, tomatoes & porcini mushrooms in the olive oil for 5- 6 minutes until softened.

**4** Add the rice and stir well for a minute or two until every grain of rice is coated with the olive oil.

**5** Add the stock and bring to the boil. Cover and place in the preheated oven for 25 minutes or until the risotto is tender and the stock has been absorbed.

**6** Check the risotto during cooking. If it needs more liquid add a little stock. If you find there is too much, remove the lid and cook for a little longer to reduce the stock.

**7** Remove from the oven, season & serve with chopped basil.

### CHEFS NOTE
You could also try some chopped sundried tomato in this veggie risotto.

# PAPRIKA POTATO GRATIN

**260**
calories per serving

## Ingredients

- 1 tbsp olive oil
- 2 onions sliced
- 800g/1¾lb potatoes, thinly sliced
- 1 tbsp paprika
- 370ml/1½ cups vegetable stock
- Salt & pepper to taste

## Method

**1** Preheat the oven to 180c/350f/Gas4

**2** Brush a flameproof casserole with the olive oil. Layer the potatoes and onions in turn in the base of the dish. Pour over the stock and sprinkle the paprika on the top.

**3** Cover and place in the oven for 1½-2 hours or until the potatoes are tender and the stock has been absorbed. Season & serve.

## CHEFS NOTE
This versatile side dish is great served with lots of freshly grated black pepper.

# BOMBAY ROAST POTATOES

**175** calories per serving

## Ingredients

- 1 tbsp olive oil
- 2 onions sliced
- 800g/1¾lb potatoes, cubed
- 1 tbsp curry powder
- Salt & pepper to taste

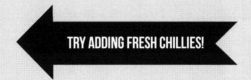

TRY ADDING FRESH CHILLIES!

## Method

**1** Preheat the oven to 180c/350f/Gas4

**2** Mix together the oil, onions, potatoes and curry powder. Place in a flameproof casserole dish or roasting tin and cook in the preheated oven for 1-1 ½ hours or until the potatoes are tender on the inside and crispy on the outside. Season & serve.

### CHEFS NOTE
Serve this side dish with some freshly chopped coriander.

# HARISSA COUSCOUS

**265** calories per serving

## Ingredients

- 1 red onion, chopped
- 2 garlic cloves, crushed
- 1 red chilli, deseeded & finely sliced
- 1 red pepper, deseeded & finely chopped
- 2 tbsp harissa paste
- 800g/1¾lb tinned chopped tomatoes
- 3 tbsp lemon juice
- 200g/7oz couscous
- 370ml/1½ cups vegetable stock
- Bunch fresh coriander/cilantro, chopped
- Low cal cooking oil spray
- Salt & pepper to taste

## Method

**1** Using a flameproof casserole dish, gently sauté the onions, garlic, chilli & peppers in a little low cal spray for a few minutes until softened (add a splash of water if it's a little dry).

**2** Add the harissa paste & chopped tomatoes, cover and leave to gently simmer for 10 minutes.

**3** Add the couscous, lemon juice and stock, remove from the heat, cover and leave for 5-10 minutes or until the couscous is tender and the stock has been reduced.

**4** Fluff the couscous with a fork, sprinkle with chopped coriander, season & serve.

### CHEFS NOTE
Harissa is an aromatic North African paste now widely available in most large food stores.

# MUSHROOM & POTATO CURRY

**290** calories per serving

## Ingredients

- 1 onion, chopped
- 500g/1lb 2oz potatoes, cubed
- 300g/11oz mushrooms, halved
- 1 red chilli, deseeded & sliced
- 2 tbsp Thai green curry paste
- 120ml/½ cup low fat coconut milk
- 120ml/½ cup vegetable stock
- 125g/4oz spinach
- Low cal cooking oil spray
- Salt & pepper to taste

## Method

**1** Using a flameproof casserole dish gently sauté the onions, potatoes, mushrooms & chillies in little low cal spray for a few minutes until softened (add a splash of water if it's a little dry).

**2** Add the curry paste, coconut milk & stock. Cover and leave to gently simmer for 10-15 minutes or until the potatoes are tender.

**3** Stir through the spinach and serve immediately.

### CHEFS NOTE
The spinach will still be fresh and crunchy if you serve immediately.

# Skinny
# ONE POT
# SEAFOOD
## DISHES

# SCOTS FISH & POTATO STEW

**460** calories per serving

## Ingredients

- 2 onions, chopped
- 800g/1¾lb potatoes, peeled & diced
- 2 tsp low fat 'butter' spread
- 500ml/2 cups semi skimmed/half fat milk
- 150g/5oz peas
- 500g/1lb 2oz boneless, smoked haddock, cubed
- Large pinch salt
- Low cal cooking oil spray
- 2 tbsp freshly chopped flat leaf parsley
- Salt & pepper to taste

## Method

**1** Using a flameproof casserole dish gently sauté the onions in a little low cal spray for a few minutes until softened (add a splash of water if it's a little dry).

**2** Add the potatoes & butter and sauté for a couple of minutes before adding the milk, peas, fish & salt. Cover and leave to gently poach for 15-20 minutes or until the fish is cooked through and the potatoes are tender.

**3** Check the stew during cooking; if it needs more liquid add some milk. Check the seasoning and serve with chopped parsley sprinkled over the top.

### CHEFS NOTE
Crush some of the potatoes with the back of a fork to thicken the sauce.

# ALMOND & FISH ONE-POT

## 340
calories per serving

## Ingredients

- 2 onions, chopped
- 2 garlic cloves, crushed
- 2 red or yellow peppers, deseeded & sliced
- 400g/14oz tinned chopped tomatoes
- 400g/14oz potatoes, peeled & cubed
- 2 tsp paprika
- 250ml/1 cup fish stock

- 2 tbsp ground almonds
- 500g/1lb 2oz boneless, white fish fillets, cubed
- Large pinch salt
- Low cal cooking oil spray
- 2 tbsp freshly chopped flat leaf parsley
- Lemon wedges to serve
- Salt & pepper to taste

## Method

**1** Using a flameproof casserole dish gently sauté the onions, garlic & peppers in a little low cal spray for a few minutes until softened (add a splash of water if it's a little dry).

**2** Add the chopped tomatoes, potatoes, paprika, stock & almonds and combine well. Cover and cook for 20 minutes, add the fish and cook for a further 10 minutes or until the fish is cooked through.

**3** Check the stew during cooking. If it needs more liquid add a little stock. If you find there is too much, remove the lid and cook for a little longer to reduce the liquid. Check the seasoning and serve with chopped parsley sprinkled over the top and lemon wedges on the side.

### CHEFS NOTE
You could use any kind of seafood you prefer in this simple stew to create a more adventurous combination.

# SHRIMP & NEW POTATO SPICY STEW

**430** calories per serving

## Ingredients

- 2 onions, chopped
- 4 slices lean, back bacon chopped
- 2 garlic cloves, crushed
- 1 red pepper, deseeded & sliced
- 1 red chilli, deseeded & sliced
- 1 tsp turmeric
- 400g/14oz tinned chopped tomatoes
- 400g/14oz new potatoes, thickly sliced

- into rounds
- 120ml/½ cup fish stock
- 120ml/½ cup white wine
- 750g/1lb 11oz peeled king prawns
- Large pinch salt
- Low cal cooking oil spray
- Salt & pepper to taste

## Method

**1** Using a flameproof casserole dish gently sauté the onions, bacon, garlic, peppers & chilli in a little low cal spray for a few minutes until softened (add a splash of water if it's a little dry).

**2** Add the turmeric, chopped tomatoes, potatoes, stock & wine and combine well. Cover and cook for 20 minutes. Add the prawns and cook for a further 10 minutes or until cooked through.

**3** Check the stew during cooking. If it needs more liquid add a little stock. If you find there is too much, remove the lid and cook for a little longer to reduce the liquid. Check the seasoning and serve.

**CHEFS NOTE**
A garnish of freshly chopped thyme makes a good addition to this dish.

# SALTED COD & CHERRY TOMATO STEW

**497** calories per serving

## Ingredients

- 1 onion, chopped, finely sliced
- 400g/14oz ripe cherry tomatoes, halved
- 2 celery stalks, chopped
- 3 garlic cloves, crushed
- 1 red pepper, deseeded & sliced
- 2 tsp paprika
- 120ml/½ cup fish stock

- 120ml/½ cup white wine
- 400g/14oz tinned butter beans, drained
- 750g/1lb 11oz pre soaked salt cod fillet, cubed
- Large pinch salt
- Low cal cooking oil spray
- Salt & pepper to taste

## Method

**1** Using a flameproof casserole dish gently sauté the onions, cherry tomatoes, celery, garlic, peppers & paprika in a little low cal spray for a few minutes until softened. (add a splash of water if it's a little dry).

**2** Add the stock and wine and leave on a medium simmer for 20 minutes, don't cover the stew as you want the liquid to reduce down.

**3** Add the butter beans and salt cod, cover and leave to gently cook for a further 10-15 minutes or until the fish is cooked through and the beans are piping hot. Check the seasoning and serve.

## CHEFS NOTE

Make sure the salt cod is properly soaked overnight in cold water.

# SEAFOOD RICE ONE-POT

**475** calories per serving

## Ingredients

- 1 onion, chopped
- 3 garlic cloves, crushed
- 50g/2oz chorizo, finely chopped
- 1 red pepper, deseeded & sliced
- ½ red chilli, deseeded & finely chopped
- 200g/7oz cherry tomatoes, halved
- 500ml/2 cups chicken or fish stock
- 200g/7oz paella rice
- Pinch of saffron strands
- 2 tbsp lemon juice
- 150g/5oz green beans, chopped
- 200g/7oz squid cleaned and sliced
- 200g/7oz shelled king prawns, chopped
- Low cal cooking oil spray
- Salt & pepper to taste

## Method

**1** Using a heavy bottomed frying pan gently sauté the onions, garlic, chorizo, peppers, chilli & cherry tomatoes in a little low cal spray for a few minutes until softened (add a splash of water if it's a little dry).

**2** Add the stock, rice, saffron & lemon juice. Bring to the boil, cover and cook for 25 minutes.

**3** Add the green beans, squid & prawns, cover and leave to simmer for a further 8-10 minutes or until the rice is tender, the stock has been absorbed and the prawns & squid are cooked through.

**4** Check the paella during cooking. If it needs more liquid add additional stock. Season and serve.

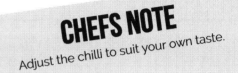

## CHEFS NOTE
Adjust the chilli to suit your own taste.

# INDIAN COD & SPINACH STEW

**390** calories per serving

## Ingredients

- 2 onions, chopped
- 2 garlic cloves, crushed
- 1 tsp freshly grated ginger
- 400g/14oz ripe cherry tomatoes, halved
- 400g/14oz potatoes, peeled & cubed
- 1 tbsp medium curry powder
- 250ml/1 cup fish or chicken stock
- 200g/7oz spinach leaves

- 600g/1lb 5oz boneless, white fish fillets, cubed
- Large pinch salt
- Low cal cooking oil spray
- 2 tbsp freshly chopped flat leaf parsley
- Lemon wedges to serve
- Salt & pepper to taste

## Method

**1** Using a flameproof casserole dish gently sauté the onions, garlic & ginger in a little low cal spray for a few minutes until softened (add a splash of water if it's a little dry).

**2** Add the cherry tomatoes, potatoes, curry powder & stock and combine well. Cook for 10 minutes on a hard simmer, add the fish and cook for a further 10 minutes or until the fish is cooked through and the potatoes are tender.

**3** Stir through the spinach for a minute or two until it is properly wilted. Check the seasoning and serve with lemon wedges on the side.

### CHEFS NOTE
Use half a teaspoon of ground ginger if you don't have fresh ginger to hand.

# SALMON & FENNEL STEW

**395** calories per serving

## Ingredients

- 2 onions, chopped
- 2 garlic cloves, crushed
- 2 carrots, finely diced
- 1 fennel bulb, finely chopped
- 3 tbsp tomato puree
- 400g/14oz potatoes, peeled & cubed
- 250ml/1 cup fish or chicken stock
- 200g/7oz green beans
- 600g/1lb 5oz boneless, salmon fillets, cubed
- Large pinch salt
- Low cal cooking oil spray
- Lemon wedges to serve
- Salt & pepper to taste

## Method

**1** Using a flameproof casserole dish gently sauté the onions, garlic, carrots & chopped fennel in a little low cal spray for a few minutes until softened (add a splash of water if it's a little dry).

**2** Add the puree, potatoes & stock and combine well. Cook for 10 minutes on a hard simmer.

**3** Add the beans & salmon, cover and leave to gently simmer for further 10 minutes or until the fish is cooked through and the potatoes are tender.

**4** Check the seasoning and serve with lemon wedges on the side.

### CHEFS NOTE
Serve this stew with lots of freshly ground black pepper.

# MUSSEL & POTATO STEW

**390** calories per serving

## Ingredients

- 2 onions, chopped
- 2 garlic cloves, crushed
- 2 carrots, finely diced
- 400g/14oz potatoes, peeled & cubed
- 100g/3½oz green beans, chopped
- 1lt/4 cups fish stock

- 1 tbsp curry powder
- 1kg/2¼lb cleaned, prepared mussels
- 120ml/½ cup low fat cream
- Low cal cooking oil spray
- Lemon wedges to serve
- Salt & pepper to taste

## Method

**1** Using a flameproof casserole dish gently sauté the onions, garlic, carrots, potatoes & green beans in a little low cal spray for approx. 10 minutes or until the potatoes are tender (add a splash of water if it's a little dry).

**2** While you are doing this bring the stock and curry powder to the boil in another pan & cook the mussels for 4-5 minutes or until their shells open. (Get rid of any mussels that don't open).

**3** Remove a ladle of stock and add to the casserole dish along with cooked mussels. Combine everything well, stir through the cream, warm for a minute or two and serve.

### CHEFS NOTE
This stew is great served with crusty bread to mop up all the creamy juices.

# MARRAKESH STEW

**483**
calories per
serving

## Ingredients

- 2 onions, chopped
- 2 garlic cloves, crushed
- 2 carrots, finely diced
- 400g/14oz tinned chopped tomatoes
- 300g/11oz tinned chickpeas, drained
- 1 tsp each turmeric, cumin & ground coriander/cilantro

- Pinch cinnamon & nutmeg
- 1 tbsp honey
- 500g/1lb 2oz shelled king prawns
- Low cal cooking oil spray
- Lemon wedges to serve
- Salt & pepper to taste

## Method

**1** Using a flameproof casserole dish gently sauté the onions, garlic & carrots in a little low cal spray for a few minutes until softened (add a splash of water if it's a little dry).

**2** Add the chopped tomatoes, chickpeas, ground spices & honey to the casserole. Combine well, cover and cook for 30 minutes.

**3** Add the prawns and gently simmer for a further 10 minutes or until the prawns are cooked through.

**4** Check the stew during cooking. If it needs more liquid add a little stock. If you find there is too much, remove the lid and cook for a little longer to reduce the liquid. Check the seasoning and serve.

**CHEFS NOTE**
Try adding some fresh chopped coriander as a garnish.

# SLOW COOKED SQUID

**390** calories per serving

## Ingredients

- 2 onions, chopped
- 2 garlic cloves, crushed
- 2 carrots, finely diced
- 800g/1¾lb tinned chopped tomatoes
- 3 tbsp tomato puree
- ½ red chilli deseeded & finely chopped
- Pinch salt & brown sugar
- 1 tsp paprika

- 1 tsp anchovy paste
- 500g/1lb 2oz prepared squid, sliced into 1cm/½ inch pieces
- 500g/1lb 2oz new potatoes, sliced
- Bunch flat leaf parsley, chopped
- Low cal cooking oil spray
- Salt & pepper to taste

## Method

**1** Using a flameproof casserole dish gently sauté the onions, garlic & carrots in a little low cal spray for a few minutes until softened (add a splash of water if it's a little dry).

**2** Add the chopped tomatoes, puree, chilli, salt, sugar, paprika & anchovy paste. Combine well, cover and cook for 10 minutes on a medium heat.

**3** After this time place the sauce in a food processor or blender and whizz until smooth. Return the blended sauce back to the casserole and add the squid. Cover and leave to gently simmer for about 50 minutes.

**4** Add the sliced new potatoes, cover and cook for a further 10-15 minute or until the potatoes are cooked through and the squid is tender.

**5** Check the stew during cooking. If it needs more liquid add a little stock. If you find there is too much, remove the lid and cook for a little longer to reduce the liquid. Check the seasoning and serve with chopped flat leaf parsley sprinkled on top.

## CHEFS NOTE

The squid should be really tender after an hour of slow cooking. Leave it to cook for longer if needed.

# MIXED SEAFOOD STEW

**295** calories per serving

## Ingredients

- 2 onions, chopped
- 2 garlic cloves, crushed
- 120ml/½ cup white wine
- 1 tsp fennel seeds
- 400g/14oz tinned chopped tomatoes
- 120ml/½ cup tomato pasatta/sauce
- ½ red chilli deseeded & finely chopped
- Pinch salt & brown sugar
- 700g/1lb 9oz mixed seafood, cubed
- Bunch fresh chopped chives
- Low cal cooking oil spray
- Salt & pepper to taste

## Method

**1** Using a flameproof casserole dish gently sauté the onions & garlic in a little low cal spray for a few minutes until softened (add a splash of water if it's a little dry). Add the wine & fennel seeds and bring to the boil. Simmer on high for 3-5 minutes or until most of the wine has reduced.

**2** Add the chopped tomatoes, passata, chilli, salt, sugar & seafood. Combine well, cover and cook for 15-20 minutes on a gentle heat.

**3** Check the seasoning and serve with chopped chives sprinkled on top.

### CHEFS NOTE
Most stores sell prepared seafood medleys which are ideal for this recipe.

# MONKFISH & MUSHROOM STEW

**285** calories per serving

## Ingredients

- 1 onion, chopped
- 2 garlic cloves, crushed
- 1 carrot, finely chopped
- 120ml/½ cup white wine
- ½ tsp fennel seeds
- 400g/14oz tinned chopped tomatoes
- 120ml/½ cup fish stock
- ½ red chilli deseeded & finely chopped
- 20g/1oz porcini mushrooms
- 200g/7oz mushrooms, sliced
- Pinch salt & brown sugar
- 700g/1lb 9oz monkfish fillets, cubed
- Low cal cooking oil spray
- Salt & pepper to taste

## Method

**1** Soak the porcini mushrooms is a little warm water for a few minutes until rehydrated, drain and finely chop.

**2** Using a flameproof casserole dish gently sauté the onions, garlic & carrots in a little low cal spray for a few minutes until softened (add a splash of water if it's a little dry).

**3** Add the wine & fennel seeds and bring to the boil. Simmer on high for 3-5 minutes until most of the wine has reduced.

**4** Add the chopped tomatoes, stock, chilli, porcini mushrooms, sliced mushrooms, salt, sugar & monkfish. Combine well, cover and cook for 30-40 minutes on a very gentle heat. Check the acidity of the tomato base and balance with a little more salt or sugar if needed.

## CHEFS NOTE

You could leave the monkfish in whole fillets if you like and serve on a bed of fresh spinach.

# ZESTY PRAWN & LEEK ONE-POT

**330**
calories per serving

## Ingredients

- 1 onion, chopped, finely sliced
- 2 leeks, finely sliced
- 400g/14oz ripe cherry tomatoes, halved
- 120ml/½ cup fish stock
- 400g/14oz tinned cannellini beans, drained
- 600g/1lb 5oz shelled king prawns
- Zest of one lemon
- Low cal cooking oil spray
- Salt & pepper to taste

## Method

**1** Using a flameproof casserole dish gently sauté the onions & leeks in a little low cal spray for a few minutes until softened (add a splash of water if it's a little dry).

**2** Add the tomatoes & fish stock, cover and cook for 40 minutes until the tomatoes break down.

**3** Add the beans & prawns, cover and leave to gently cook for a further 10 minutes or until the prawns are cooked through and the beans are piping hot.

**4** Stir through the lemon zest, check the seasoning and serve.

### CHEFS NOTE
Use meaty white fish fillets instead of prawns if you prefer.

# SUPER QUICK TUNA 'STEW' ON TOAST

**430** calories per serving

## Ingredients

- 1 onion, finely sliced
- 100g/3½oz pitted black olives, halved
- ½ tsp brown sugar
- 600g/1lb 5oz fresh tuna steak, cut into strips
- 5 large vine ripened tomatoes, roughly chopped
- 60ml/¼ cup fish stock
- 60ml/¼ cup soy sauce
- 4 slices thick granary bread, light toasted
- Low cal cooking oil spray
- Salt & pepper to taste

## Method

1 Using a frying pan gently sauté the onion, olives & sugar in a little low cal spray for a few minutes until softened (add a splash of water to the pan if it's a little dry).

2 Add the tuna, tomatoes, stock & soy sauce, combine well and cook for 4-6 minutes or until the tuna is cooked through.

3 Check the seasoning and serve on top of the toasted granary bread.

### CHEFS NOTE
A tablespoon of chopped capers makes a great addition to this super-quick stew.

# PRAWN & SQUASH ASIAN ONE-POT

**295** calories per serving

## Ingredients

- 2 onions, chopped
- 2 garlic cloves, crushed
- 1 butternut squash, peeled, deseeded & cubed
- 1 tbsp fish sauce
- 1 tbsp Thai red curry paste
- 1 tbsp lime pickle

- 120ml/½ cup low fat coconut milk
- 200g/7oz green beans
- 600g/1lb 5oz shelled, king prawns
- Low cal cooking oil spray
- Lemon wedges to serve
- Salt & pepper to taste

## Method

**1** Using a flameproof casserole dish gently sauté the onions, garlic & chopped squash in a little low cal spray for a few minutes until softened (add a splash of water if it's a little dry).

**2** Add the fish sauce, curry paste, lime pickle & coconut milk. Cover and gently simmer for 20 minutes. Add the green beans & prawns, cover and leave to gently simmer for a further 10 minutes or until the prawns are cooked through and the squash is tender.

**3** Check the seasoning and serve.

### CHEFS NOTE
This stew is lovely served with rice or noodles and chopped coriander.

# SPANISH SEAFOOD RISOTTO

**450** calories per serving

## Ingredients

- 1 tbsp olive oil
- 1 red pepper, deseeded & sliced
- 1 onion, chopped
- 2 garlic cloves, crushed
- 250g/9oz risotto rice

- 750g/3 cups vegetable stock
- 2 tsp paprika
- 1 tsp turmeric
- 400g/14oz shelled prawns, chopped
- Salt & pepper to taste

## Method

**1** Preheat the oven to 180c/350f/Gas4

**2** Using a flameproof casserole dish gently sauté the peppers, onion & garlic in the olive oil for about 5 minutes until softened.

**3** Add the rice and stir well for a minute or two until every grain of rice is coated with the olive oil.

**4** Add the stock, paprika & turmeric and bring to the boil. Cover and place in the preheated oven for 15 minutes. Add the prawns, return to the oven and cook for 10-15 minutes or until the risotto is tender, the stock has been absorbed and the prawns are cooked through.

**5** Check the risotto during cooking. If it needs more liquid add a little stock. If you find there is too much, remove the lid and cook for a little longer to reduce the stock.

**6** Remove from the oven, season & serve.

## CHEFS NOTE

You could also add some chopped chorizo to this Spanish dish.

# OVEN BAKED KEDGEREE

**400**
calories per serving

## Ingredients

- 1 onion, chopped
- 2 garlic cloves, crushed
- 1 tsp turmeric
- 200g/7oz long grain rice
- 150g/5oz peas
- 750ml/3 cups fish or chicken stock
- 400g/14oz smoked haddock, cut into chunks

- 4 hardboiled eggs, chopped
- Bunch spring onions/scallions, chopped
- Bunch flat leaf parsley, chopped
- Low cal cooking oil spray
- Salt & pepper to taste

## Method

**1** Preheat the oven to 180c/350f/Gas4

**2** Using a flameproof casserole dish gently sauté the onions & garlic in a little low cal spray for a few minutes until the onions are softened (add a splash of water if it's a little dry).

**3** Add the turmeric, rice, peas & stock and cook for a few minutes. Add the beans & stock. Cover and place in the preheated oven for 10 minutes.

**4** Add the haddock and combine well. Cover and cook for a further 10-15 minutes or until the haddock is cooked through, the rice is tender and the stock has been absorbed.

**5** Check the kedgeree during cooking. If it needs more liquid add a little stock. If you find there is too much, remove the lid and cook for a little longer to reduce the liquid.

**6** Meanwhile mix together the chopped eggs, spring onion & parsley. When the kedgeree is cooked stir the egg and onion mixture through the rice. Season and serve.

### CHEFS NOTE
Try adding a little paprika to the egg & onion mixture.

# Skinny
# ONE POT
# STOCK

Homemade stock is not essential, but if you would like to try making your own, you will find it can add additional depth of taste and further improve the flavour of some dishes. Having said that, store-bought stock has vastly improved in recent times and you may well decide making your own stock isn't worth the time for the comparable result. If you do use store-bought stock (which most people do) avoid buying budget options and anything too high in sodium.

# BASIC VEGETABLE STOCK

## Ingredients

- Ingredients:
- 1 tbsp olive oil
- 1 onion, chopped
- 1 leek, chopped
- 1 carrot, chopped
- 1 small bulb fennel, chopped
- 3 garlic cloves, crushed
- 1 tbsp black peppercorns
- 75g/3oz mushrooms
- 2 sticks celery, chopped
- 3 tomatoes, diced
- 2 tbsp freshly chopped flat leaf parsley
- 2 bay leaves
- 3lt/12 cups water

## Method

1 Gently sauté the onions, leeks, carrots and fennel in the olive oil for a few minutes in a large lidded saucepan.

2 Add all the other ingredients, cover and bring to the boil. Leave to gently simmer for 20 minutes with the lid on.

3 Allow to cool for a little while. Pour the contents through a sieve and store the finished stock liquid in the fridge for a couple of days or freeze in batches.

# BASIC CHICKEN STOCK

## Ingredients

- 1 tbsp olive oil
- 1 left over roast chicken carcass
- 2 carrots, chopped
- 2 onions, halved
- 2 stalks celery, chopped

- 10 black peppercorns
- 2 bay leaves
- 2 tbsp freshly chopped parsley
- 1 tsp freshly chopped thyme
- 3lt/12 cups water

## Method

**1** Gently sauté the onions, carrots and celery in the olive oil for a few minutes in a large lidded saucepan.

**2** Break the chicken carcass up into pieces and add to the pan along with all the other ingredients, cover and bring to the boil. Leave on a very gentle simmer for 1hr with the lid on. Allow to cool for a little while.

**3** Pour the contents through a sieve and store the finished stock liquid in the fridge for a couple of days or freeze in batches. You may find you need to skim a little fat from the top of the stock after cooking.

# BASIC BEEF STOCK

## Ingredients

- 1 tbsp olive oil
- 1kg/2¼lb beef bones
- 3 carrots, chopped
- 3 onions, halved

- 10 black peppercorns
- 2 bay leaves
- 2 tbsp freshly chopped parsley
- 3.5lt/14 cups water

## Method

**1** Gently sauté the onions and carrots in the olive oil for a few minutes in a large lidded saucepan.

**2** Add the beef bones to the pan along with all the other ingredients, cover and bring to the boil. Leave on a very gentle simmer for 1hr-2hrs with the lid on.

**3** Allow to cool for a little while. Pour the contents through a sieve and store the finished stock liquid in the fridge for a couple of days or freeze in batches. You may find you need to skim a little fat from the top of the stock after cooking.

# BASIC FISH STOCK

## Ingredients

- 1 tbsp olive oil
- 450g/1lb fish bones, heads carcasses etc (avoid oily fish when making stock)
- 4 leeks, chopped
- 1 fennel bulb, chopped
- 4 carrots, chopped
- 2 tbsp freshly chopped parsley
- 250ml/1 cup dry white wine
- 2.5lt/10 cups water

## Method

**1** Gently sauté the carrots, leeks and fennel in the olive oil for a few minutes in a large lidded saucepan.

**2** Clean the fish bones to ensure there is no blood as this can 'spoil' the stock. Add all the other ingredients, cover and bring to the boil. Leave on a very gentle simmer for 1hr with the lid on.

**3** Allow to cool for a little while. Pour the contents through a sieve and store the finished stock liquid in the fridge for a couple of days or freeze in batches. You may find you need to skim a little fat from the top of the stock after cooking.

# Other
# COOKNATION
# TITLES

If you enjoyed 'The Skinny One Pot, Casseroles & Stews Recipe Book' we'd really appreciate your feedback. Reviews help others decide if this is the right book for them.

# Thank you.

You may also be interested in other '**Skinny**' titles in the CookNation series. You can find all the following great titles by searching under '**CookNation**'.

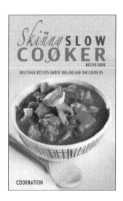

## THE SKINNY SLOW COOKER RECIPE BOOK

Delicious Recipes Under 300, 400 And 500 Calories.

**Paperback / eBook**

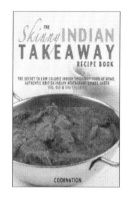

## THE SKINNY INDIAN TAKEAWAY RECIPE BOOK

Authentic British Indian Restaurant Dishes Under 300, 400 And 500 Calories. The Secret To Low Calorie Indian Takeaway Food At Home.

**Paperback / eBook**

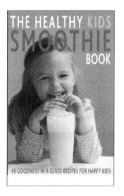

## THE HEALTHY KIDS SMOOTHIE BOOK

40 Delicious Goodness In A Glass Recipes for Happy Kids.

**eBook**

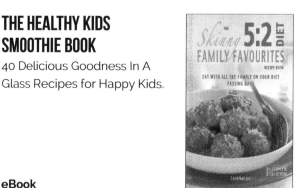

## THE SKINNY 5:2 FAST DIET FAMILY FAVOURITES RECIPE BOOK

Eat With All The Family On Your Diet Fasting Days.

**Paperback / eBook**

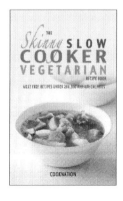

## THE SKINNY SLOW COOKER VEGETARIAN RECIPE BOOK

40 Delicious Recipes Under 200, 300 And 400 Calories.

**Paperback / eBook**

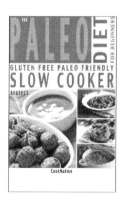

## THE PALEO DIET FOR BEGINNERS SLOW COOKER RECIPE BOOK

Gluten Free, Everyday Essential Slow Cooker Paleo Recipes For Beginners.

**eBook**

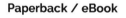

## THE SKINNY 5:2 SLOW COOKER RECIPE BOOK

Skinny Slow Cooker Recipe And Menu Ideas Under 100, 200, 300 & 400 Calories For Your 5:2 Diet.

**Paperback / eBook**

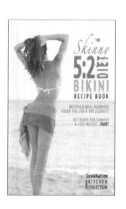

## THE SKINNY 5:2 BIKINI DIET RECIPE BOOK

Recipes & Meal Planners Under 100, 200 & 300 Calories. Get Ready For Summer & Lose Weight...FAST!

**Paperback / eBook**

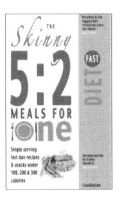

### THE SKINNY 5:2 FAST DIET MEALS FOR ONE

Single Serving Fast Day Recipes & Snacks Under 100, 200 & 300 Calories.

**Paperback / eBook**

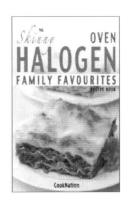

### THE SKINNY HALOGEN OVEN FAMILY FAVOURITES RECIPE BOOK

Healthy, Low Calorie Family Meal-Time Halogen Oven Recipes Under 300, 400 and 500 Calories.

**Paperback / eBook**

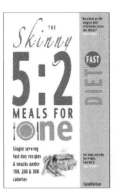

### THE SKINNY 5:2 FAST DIET VEGETARIAN MEALS FOR ONE

Single Serving Fast Day Recipes & Snacks Under 100, 200 & 300 Calories.

**Paperback / eBook**

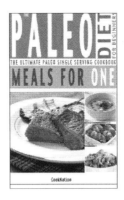

### THE PALEO DIET FOR BEGINNERS MEALS FOR ONE

The Ultimate Paleo Single Serving Cookbook.

**Paperback / eBook**

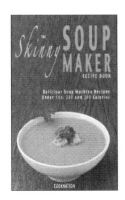

### THE SKINNY SOUP MAKER RECIPE BOOK

Delicious Low Calorie, Healthy and Simple Soup Recipes Under 100, 200 and 300 Calories. Perfect For Any Diet and Weight Loss Plan.

**Paperback / eBook**

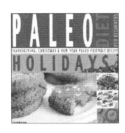

### THE PALEO DIET FOR BEGINNERS HOLIDAYS

Thanksgiving, Christmas & New Year Paleo Friendly Recipes.
**eBook**

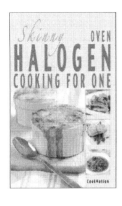

### SKINNY HALOGEN OVEN COOKING FOR ONE

Single Serving, Healthy, Low Calorie Halogen Oven RecipesUnder 200, 300 and 400 Calories.

**Paperback / eBook**

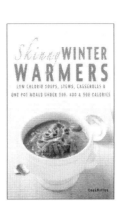

### SKINNY WINTER WARMERS RECIPE BOOK

Soups, Stews, Casseroles & One Pot Meals Under 300, 400 & 500 Calories.

**Paperback / eBook**

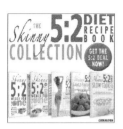

## THE SKINNY 5:2 DIET RECIPE BOOK COLLECTION

All The 5:2 Fast Diet Recipes You'll Ever Need. All Under 100, 200, 300, 400 And 500 Calories.

**eBook**

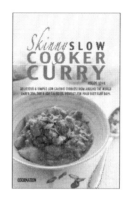

## THE SKINNY SLOW COOKER CURRY RECIPE BOOK

Low Calorie Curries From Around The World.

**Paperback / eBook**

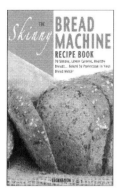

## THE SKINNY BREAD MACHINE RECIPE BOOK

70 Simple, Lower Calorie, Healthy Breads...Baked To Perfection In Your Bread Maker.

**Paperback / eBook**

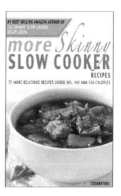

## MORE SKINNY SLOW COOKER RECIPES

75 More Delicious Recipes Under 300, 400 & 500 Calories.

**Paperback / eBook**

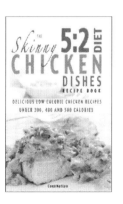

## THE SKINNY 5:2 DIET CHICKEN DISHES RECIPE BOOK

Delicious Low Calorie Chicken Dishes Under 300, 400 & 500 Calories.

**Paperback / eBook**

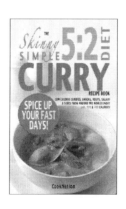

## THE SKINNY 5:2 CURRY RECIPE BOOK

Spice Up Your Fast Days With Simple Low Calorie Curries, Snacks, Soups, Salads & Sides Under 200, 300 & 400 Calories.

**Paperback / eBook**

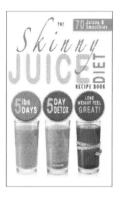

## THE SKINNY JUICE DIET RECIPE BOOK

5lbs, 5 Days. The Ultimate Kick- Start Diet and Detox Plan to Lose Weight & Feel Great!

**Paperback / eBook**

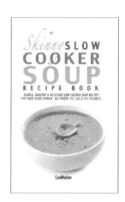

## THE SKINNY SLOW COOKER SOUP RECIPE BOOK

Simple, Healthy & Delicious Low Calorie Soup Recipes For Your Slow Cooker. All Under 100, 200 & 300 Calories.

**Paperback / eBook**

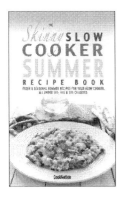

## THE SKINNY SLOW COOKER SUMMER RECIPE BOOK

Fresh & Seasonal Summer Recipes For Your Slow Cooker. All Under 300, 400 And 500 Calories.

**Paperback / eBook**

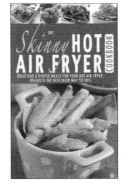

## THE SKINNY HOT AIR FRYER COOKBOOK

Delicious & Simple Meals For Your Hot Air Fryer: Discover The Healthier Way To Fry.

**Paperback / eBook**

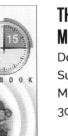

## THE SKINNY ACTIFRY COOKBOOK

Guilt-free and Delicious ActiFry Recipe Ideas: Discover The Healthier Way to Fry!

**Paperback / eBook**

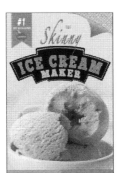

## THE SKINNY ICE CREAM MAKER

Delicious Lower Fat, Lower Calorie Ice Cream, Frozen Yogurt & Sorbet Recipes For Your Ice Cream Maker.

**Paperback / eBook**

## THE SKINNY 15 MINUTE MEALS RECIPE BOOK

Delicious, Nutritious & Super-Fast Meals in 15 Minutes Or Less. All Under 300, 400 & 500 Calories.

**Paperback / eBook**

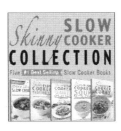

## THE SKINNY SLOW COOKER COLLECTION

5 Fantastic Books of Delicious, Diet-friendly Skinny Slow Cooker Recipes: ALL Under 200, 300, 400 & 500 Calories!
**eBook**

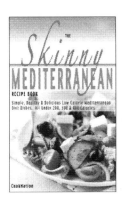

## THE SKINNY MEDITERRANEAN RECIPE BOOK

Simple, Healthy & Delicious Low Calorie Mediterranean Diet Dishes. All Under 200, 300 & 400 Calories.

**Paperback / eBook**

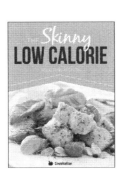

## THE SKINNY LOW CALORIE RECIPE BOOK

Great Tasting, Simple & Healthy Meals Under 300, 400 & 500 Calories. Perfect For Any Calorie Controlled Diet.

**Paperback / eBook**

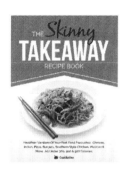

## THE SKINNY TAKEAWAY RECIPE BOOK

Healthier Versions Of Your Fast Food Favourites: All Under 300, 400 & 500 Calories.

**Paperback / eBook**

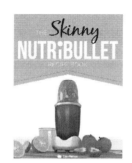

## THE SKINNY NUTRIBULLET RECIPE BOOK

80+ Delicious & Nutritious Healthy Smoothie Recipes. Burn Fat, Lose Weight and Feel Great!

**Paperback / eBook**

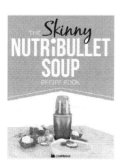

## THE SKINNY NUTRIBULLET SOUP RECIPE BOOK

Delicious, Quick & Easy, Single Serving Soups & Pasta Sauces For Your Nutribullet. All Under 100, 200, 300 & 400 Calories!

**Paperback / eBook**

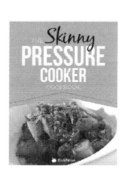

## THE SKINNY PRESSURE COOKER COOKBOOK

*USA ONLY*
Low Calorie, Healthy & Delicious Meals, Sides & Desserts. All Under 300, 400 & 500 Calories.

**Paperback / eBook**

# CONVERSION CHART: DRY INGREDIENTS

| Metric | Imperial |
|--------|----------|
| 7g | ¼ oz |
| 15g | ½ oz |
| 20g | ¾ oz |
| 25g | 1 oz |
| 40g | 1½oz |
| 50g | 2oz |
| 60g | 2½oz |
| 75g | 3oz |
| 100g | 3½oz |
| 125g | 4oz |
| 140g | 4½oz |
| 150g | 5oz |
| 165g | 5½oz |
| 175g | 6oz |
| 200g | 7oz |
| 225g | 8oz |
| 250g | 9oz |
| 275g | 10oz |
| 300g | 11oz |
| 350g | 12oz |
| 375g | 13oz |
| 400g | 14oz |

| Metric | Imperial |
|--------|----------|
| 425g | 15oz |
| 450g | 1lb |
| 500g | 1lb 2oz |
| 550g | 1¼lb |
| 600g | 1lb 5oz |
| 650g | 1lb 7oz |
| 675g | 1½lb |
| 700g | 1lb 9oz |
| 750g | 1lb 11oz |
| 800g | 1¾lb |
| 900g | 2lb |
| 1kg | 2¼lb |
| 1.1kg | 2½lb |
| 1.25kg | 2¾lb |
| 1.35kg | 3lb |
| 1.5kg | 3lb 6oz |
| 1.8kg | 4lb |
| 2kg | 4½lb |
| 2.25kg | 5lb |
| 2.5kg | 5½lb |
| 2.75kg | 6lb |

# CONVERSION CHART: LIQUID MEASURES

| Metric | Imperial | US |
|--------|----------|------|
| 25ml | 1fl oz | |
| 60ml | 2fl oz | ¼ cup |
| 75ml | 2½ fl oz | |
| 100ml | 3½fl oz | |
| 120ml | 4fl oz | ½ cup |
| 150ml | 5fl oz | |
| 175ml | 6fl oz | |
| 200ml | 7fl oz | |
| 250ml | 8½ fl oz | 1 cup |
| 300ml | 10½ fl oz | |
| 360ml | 12½ fl oz | |
| 400ml | 14fl oz | |
| 450ml | 15½ fl oz | |
| 600ml | 1 pint | |
| 750ml | 1¼ pint | 3 cups |
| 1 litre | 1½ pints | 4 cups |

Printed in Great Britain
by Amazon